# OBTAINABLE

Enjoy the Body and Energy You've Always Wanted –
Beyond Diet and Exercise

Cover by StoryBuilders —MyStoryBuilders.com

This book is dedicated to my lovely bride Dari. Without her, my life would be far too crazy for me to handle. She gives me balance, perspective, and hope. I love you.

**OBTAINABLE – ENJOY THE BODY AND ENERGY YOU'VE ALWAYS WANTED – BEYOND DIET AND EXERCISE**

Copyright © 2019 by Warren Willey
Published by StoryBuilders & The Fitness Medicine Clinic
Pocatello, Idaho 83201
ISBN# 9781729535882

ALL RIGHTS RESERVED. No part of this publication may be reproduced, stored in a retrieval system, or transmitted in any form or by any means – electronic, mechanical, digital, photocopy, recording, or any other – except for brief quotations in printed reviews, without the prior written permission of Dr. Willey.

Hey! Don't you know it's a waste of your day…?
Caught up in endless solutions,
That have no meaning, just another hunch based upon jumping conclusions…
Caught up in endless solutions…
Backed up against a wall of confusion…
Living a life of illusion…

—Joe Walsh

"All truth passes through three stages: first, it is ridiculed. Second, it is violently opposed. Third, it is accepted as self-evident."

—Arthur Schopenhauer

***\*** WARNING: This book is not a quick fix. If you needed results yesterday, put this book down and save it for when you have more time, or finally give in to the realization that nothing you are doing is working. *****

# TABLE OF CONTENTS

Preface ............................................................................................ ix

## PART I. THE FAT TO FIT TO FAT PROGRAM .......... 1

### Chapter 1: Change Your Body, Change Your Life? ............... 3
- Categories of Physique Obtaining Programs ....................... 7
- How Often Do Modern Diet and Exercise Plans work? ......... 7
- The After Picture .................................................. 8

### Chapter 2: Don't Blame Me! ................................................. 11
- Personal Revelation into the Calorie Myth ........................ 19
- Fat is Adaptive .................................................... 24

### Chapter 3: Case Studies of People Just Like You ................... 29
- The Once-Upon-a-Time Bodybuilder ............................... 32
- The Fitness Girl ................................................... 40
- The Yo-Yo ......................................................... 47
- Up 20+ Pounds in Menopause ..................................... 52
- The Ex-College Athlete (as told by her) .......................... 55
- For the Long Haul ................................................. 60
- My Classic Patient (as told by my medical assistant) .......... 64

## PART II. SUMMARY OF MODERN DIET AND EXERCISE PROGRAMS AND THEIR PROBLEMS .. 69

### Chapter 4: Problem 1—Too Much Exercise ............................ 73

### Chapter 5: Problem 2—Too Little Eating (or) Get the Body I Want NOW Eating ......................................................... 83

### Chapter 6: Problem 3—The Supplements and the Drugs ........... 99

Chapter 7: Diets Written Under the Guise of Medical Supervision .................................................................. 115

# PART III—THE FIX

Chapter 8: The Medical Evaluation ................................................. 128

Chapter 9: *RecoverMe* Exercise ....................................................... 177

Chapter 10: *RecoverMe* Eating ........................................................ 229

Chapter 11: *RecoverMe* Suggested Supplements ......................... 277

Chapter 12: *RecoverMe* Sleep ......................................................... 293

Chapter 13: Conclusions and FAQs ................................................ 325

Appendix I: The Willey Principle .......................................................... 347

Appendix II: Protein Sources with Grams Per Serving Size ............. 351

Appendix III: Meditation and Sauna Use ............................................ 355

Contact Information ............................................................................... 359

Index .......................................................................................................... 361

# PREFACE

This book is devoted to anyone and everyone who has ever attempted to lose weight, obtain a desired physique or look, or has lost weight only to find it come back. This is a big audience. I felt it important to include those people too who have ever done a physique show, done athletics (high school, college, or professional) but are now "stuck" with a body that is not cooperating with them. It is difficult going from a lean mean machine at one time to someone who cannot get back into shape, no matter what is done or attempted. This book will explain how you got there and how to potentially get it back.

There is an incredible need for this information as my contemporaries and I are seeing more and more problems with contemporary diet and exercise recommendations in our medical practices. It is not always apparent that the issue being presented has a direct correlation with the aspiration, possibly a preconceived need, to obtain a desired look. Hence, the information provided in this book—it's for my colleagues as well.

When I lecture, I often allude to the fallacy of modern diet and exercise programs. I am often asked how current diet and exercise recommendations have failed. That question is almost universally followed with the statement "I thought diet and exercise were good for me." My response is always in the positive, within limits. Yes, they are good for you when done correctly. Yes, they are good for you if you can control all the other stress variables in your life. Yes, they are good for you if you recover well from the diet and exercise recommendations. It is false to assume that all the diet and exercise programs available are out to see you improve your quality of life. They provide you with a set standard and goal to strive for, usually a number such as your scale weight, and provide you a temporary means of reaching it, without any forethought on long-term consequences. What modern diet and exercise suggestions do to your body is quite shocking, as it is about everything you would not have anticipated. This truth needs exposure.

Part of the extreme push toward these diet and exercise programs, as well as the weekly fad program that appears on the Internet, is due to the fact we are a society of images. Images of the perfect body, both male and female, are everywhere. From social media outlets, to superhero movies, cartoons for kids, advertisements for toilet paper—you cannot escape these images. These images are burned into your mind, and many a person's entire life goal starts to focus on becoming one of these images. Any variation of this assumed perfection is ridiculed, and assumptions are made about health, happiness, and quality of life. It is a vicious spiral downward into depression and poor health as the method being professed to obtain that look is dangerous.

The entire weight loss industry has completely, not necessarily innocently, missed the boat on how real body composition changes can and do occur. The professed "calories-in-to-calories-out" also known as "eat less, exercise more" approach is actually part of the problem. It's starting to come to light, and this book was written to be a beacon for people struggling with their body composition and health, no matter what their background.

What is becoming so blatantly apparent is that eating less and less while exercising more and more is really causing fat gain, increasing disease, and decreasing the quality of life, not improving it.

The question arises then as to why it is so hard to maintain the Adonis or Aphrodite look? Or for those who never got it when they were after it, why was it insurmountable? How could anyone exercise so hard, eat so well, and still not get there? Some of the most frustrated people I have ever worked with fit this bill. They really are trying, but nothing is working. I hope to answer that question in this little book. More importantly, I hope to show you how to get past it and achieve a degree of body refinement that is maintainable for life.

    I have kept it short and to the point. I am the king of esoteric, and I love to read, then talk about, everything I can get my hands on. That does not describe most people these days. Our attention spans are no longer than our arms. We love *short* videos, images, and the last thing we want to see is too much detail. "Get to the point, Doctor!" is something I know my patients are thinking quite often. I will with this book. I am going to get to the point, keep it short, keep you entertained, and hopefully help you learn something about these programs out there, and a little about yourself and your health in the process. In doing so, I will not be listing references. I have them if you want them, but having written several books, deciding what references to list, listing them correctly for my high-school English teacher, and finding space for them in the book are all too painful. If you want more detail on any part or section, email me.

    The original title of this book was **Fat to Fit to Fat**. As I was the only one that really understood the implications of that title, I changed it to avoid confusion. All current diet and exercise recommendations cause your fat to go away (at least the first time you do it), get you in some kind of shape, then your fat comes back on with a vengeance. What I am implying is that doing one of these modern programs, be it the exercise or diet, does really nothing to your fatness or health, other than temporarily appear to change it. It is still there, you just think it's gone. Do you know why I know that? I understand the physiology behind this type of diet. Do you know why *you* know it to be true? Quit the programs and see what happens.

    I will be referring to these flawed modern diet and exercise programs throughout the book and I hope to explain why they are defective. I will occasionally call them Fat to Fit programs because I could not completely abandon the name as it is so applicable.

Admittedly, I do not have a ton of "evidence-based" data to back what I am telling you here. As a physician, I am overly aware that we all conform ourselves to the wisdom of our own decisions—"That person got better after seeing me because of my intervention." In reality, and in a large number of cases of illness, they would have gotten better on their own without my interference. In medicine, to acknowledge uncertainty is to confess to the possibility of error. I am probably guilty of exaggerated confidence based on my experience. That being said (and humor intended), what I am about to tell you in this book works. Would most people feel better, have a higher quality of life if they just quit trying so hard and working so hard for that perfect body? Yes, of course. Can the information in this book help you get there quicker AND help you achieve the body you want? Once again, yes. It can.

## A Little Background

It is probably important for me to provide you with some background on why I wrote this book, and why I likely qualify for writing this book.

I am a practicing physician in Southeast Idaho, and I am blessed with a worldwide patient selection. People fly in from all over the United States and the world to visit with me regarding optimal health, weight loss, a unique approach to their chronic disease, and physique morphing. I have a great practice, as most of the people I see really want to live optimally. People with a quality of life goal tend to do better with instructions and following directions.

I don't advertise or proclaim a lot on social media as I enjoy my quiet life. I am starting to do more social media at the nudging of my business partners and marketing staff, but don't expect too much. My name has gotten out there due to a few books I have written and the wonderful opportunities I have had to talk with doctors around the country while lecturing at medical conferences. Again, never advertising anything, two books in particular just slowly grew. The first one was **What Does Your Doctor Look Like Naked?**—a book I started in the 1990s about optimal health, antiaging, and what we now call functional medicine. It, by the way, is the namesake of this book and a series of books following.

The second book that developed sort of a cult following was **Better Than Steroids**, endorsed by Mr. Olympia at the time, Jay Cutler. It is all about utilizing dietary techniques to obtain the physique you have always wanted. It works well and, although I did not add all the eating plans we utilized back then (some of which I talk about here in this book), its information is ageless, and I still get a few emails a day, twelve years after its publication, with questions and praises.

I tell you this as that is what set me up for seeing the wonderful clients I see today. I get to see everyone from professional athletes to 80-year-old women who just want to feel better and have more energy (believe it or not, there are a lot of similarities between these two—what most would consider opposite poles).

I do what others would call functional medicine but have been doing it for years before the term came about. I like the term, as it is applicable—Western medicine is more compartmental or anatomical, whereas the body is an intertwined, functional unit that is very sensitive to outside influences.

I am board-certified with The American Board of Antiaging/Regenerative Medicine, The American Board of Obesity Medicine, and The American Board of Family Medicine. I love to focus on body optimization including diet and exercise and hormones—as they control everything. I coined the term "Bariatric Endocrinology" to describe what I do, but I like to consider myself a "*Commonsenseist*" (like a proctologist, but different): Optimize what crosses your lips, move as often as you can, be aware of and avoid toxins in your environment—if you are exposed, learn how to deal with them, help your body manage stress, consider the spiritual aspects of your being, and enjoy life until the Good Lord says you're done. That is what I do.

I utilize dietary measures based on hormonal response, exercise or movement instructions based on hormonal response, individualized supplement programs, hormonal optimization with prescriptions and/or diet/supplements, and other medications, as needed. I joke with people all the time that I am a legal drug dealer, just not a drug pusher. Medications have their place, but one gets to that place, in most cases, by lifestyle choices and environmental effects, not by bad luck, or genetics.

Helping people do bodybuilding shows for the last 30+ years, I have amassed a database that has allowed me to look back and see trends, what

> "Getting ready for a bodybuilding show" could easily be substituted with "Going on a diet" or "Doing a 12-week biggest loser contest," etc.

works, what does not work, etc. Hence this book—I started to see the absolute long-term failure of "getting ready for a bodybuilding show" years ago, but the programs worked in the short run (people like me could get almost anyone ready for a show, but then what?), so we all kept writing them. After all, if someone got fat after doing a show it was their fault, right?

This practice means I have a lot of people coming to me who want to do physique shows and people who want to lose weight. At the risk of sounding boastful, I can do that, and do it well—but my first goal for anyone with that wish is their overall health and long-term well-being. Unless the bodybuilding or a fitness show diet is done correctly, *slowly* (not 12 weeks or any other short-term random number), and with long-term plans in mind, people rebound hard. I cannot tell you the number of times I have seen that. It is heartbreaking for me to see people obtain an optimal physique and then lose it. It is even more heartbreaking to them, I am sure. I also have a heart for all the people I see in the gym, exercising very hard, but either not changing or getting fatter. Something is up, and that "up" is the fact that they are following a modern diet and exercise program I will describe here.

My hope is that while reading (or hearing) this book, you will have the tools to change your lifestyle and start pursuing long-term goals and plans. Take the slow burn to physique optimization, weight loss, health obtainment, and really lead the good life. Get off the eat less and exercise more train, and do it correctly—finally!

I have so many people to thank that were involved in the groundwork for this book, I could never list them all. My good friend and business partner Randy Vawdrey NP-C and his incredible insight into the real cause of disease, my copyeditor Nancy Wall, proofreaders and content modifiers—my wonderful wife Dari, Penny Pink, Trilby Wedler, Jared Barton, Marci Barnes, Katlynn Hudson, and the many people I suckered into reading the book—occasionally just scattered chapters at a time. They acted as my focus group, making a complex topic more accessible. A heartfelt thank you!

As a lot of the content here is likely to raise questions or get you wondering about your own state of health, I have left my contact information at the end of the book. I am more than happy to help you if I can, or at least suggest someone in your area who may be able to help you. If you are interested in the slow burn and want to approach it on your own, take the information you have learned in this book and start by watching my YouTube channel: https://www.youtube.com/user/DrWilleydotcom

I have many 2–4-minute videos that sum up the healthy lifestyle that makes a big difference in the long run. You could also check out my **What Does Your Doctor Look Like Naked?** book series—it's a reprint and collection of all my books. It comes with access to online support, blogs, and a community of people who have found, hopefully like you after reading this book, that they have been shamed by the Fat to Fit programs out there and there is a way to fix what has been damaged. These can be ordered at www.drwilley.com.

Enough said; let us get started.

# PART I
## The Fat to Fit to Fat Program

- Chapter 1: Change Your Body, Change Your Life?
- Chapter 2: Don't Blame Me!
- Chapter 3: Case Studies of People Just Like You

# CHAPTER 1
## Change Your Body, Change Your Life?

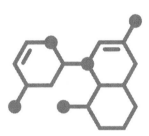

I think it's Gold's Gym that copyrighted the phrase "Change your body, change your life." Their entire premise and approach to "changing your body" is part of the problem with weight issues and disease states related to weight problems in this country. Not to mention the psychological damage and the incredible rise in depression, anxiety, sleep issues, increase in disability claims, and even frank psychosis. Is it a stretch for me to blame these disease states on the premise behind this statement? No, it's not. Especially when you understand that what others may call disease states, are simply symptoms of underlying issues related to lifestyle choices.

The premise behind the statement "Change your body, change your life" is you need to exercise a lot to get the body you want. Implicit in that definition is the fact you need to cut your calories and eat less as well (whatever that means).

Eating correctly and exercising are of course good for you. In and of themselves they are a part of a proper lifestyle program that keeps you healthy and with a good, long, quality of life. It's the intensity and/or amount of exercise alongside extremes of caloric restriction under a given time frame that can cause serious issues and illness. This has never really been considered before.

This scenario plays out in many different presentations from gut issues, to brain issues, to sexual issues, to severe fatigue, to hormonal issues—a reason why I wrote this book. This book's strategy is to make you aware of all the things that go wrong when you com-bine the stress of everyday, modern, high-tech, demanding living, and add vigorous exercise and restrictive dieting to it. In one form or another, in one way or another, it will catch up to you if you are not aware of it.

The "modern dieting" approach of extreme exercise and limited eating causes a ton of stress on the body and causes more issues than you are likely cognizant of. One you are most certainly familiar with is the severe rebound weight gain after a modern dietary or exercise program. This includes the big national programs that supply all your "food" for you, the DVD set you bought on late night television that invites you to torture yourself in the comforts of your own living room, the popular cable programs that show others in extremes of pain and agony doing the same thing. Modern dieting and exercise cause an underlying damage to your hormones, your gut, increase oxidative stress, expose you to toxins, and cause an array of symptoms that most doctors will just attribute to depression or some other underlying psychiatric illness.

Of course, there is an entire population that gets sick, feels horrible, and has a poor quality of life because they do not move, and they do not watch what goes in their mouths. They are also those who are exposed to toxins and environmental influences that have devastating consequences and their bodies are not able to handle it as others may be inclined to do. ***I am not writing this book for them.***

This book is for everyone who tries their best to exercise and eat right using the modern dietary misconceptions described here.

The problem with contemporary diet and exercise recommendations is universal and becoming more of a problem as more and more people are trying to get new bodies. Everyone is on the bandwagon and no one is questioning its validity.

As far as people using this misinformation to change their physique are concerned, I often ask why am I seeing this more than ever before, being in the health and fitness industry for over 35 years. This could be because of social media and the Internet, as we have become an image society. Everyone thinks that having a certain look is the only way to happiness. I have a few other ideas as to why it is so prevalent, but this is not the forum to discuss them. I can tell you that back in the 1980s when I started my venture in the physique world, people even going to health clubs were few and far between! The fitness magazines had real articles, not advertisements. The only advertisements they had were for gym equipment, as there were very few health clubs at the time! Tangent. Sorry, let's get back to the reason I wrote this book. I wrote it to help many people who are suffering from the same problem, even though their backgrounds are different. These people can be summed up in six categories:

1. The man or woman who, at one time, trained hard and got into contest/stage shape did do a physique show, a bodybuilding show, or a fitness show. Following it, they lost all their gains and cannot get that body back.

2. A similar person as those above who, no matter what they do, cannot get into bodybuilding, physique, or fitness shape.

3. The ex-college or professional athletes who after retiring from playing sports lost all their lean mass and replaced it with fat, against their will.

4. The people who cannot lose weight no matter how hard they try, including the good people who used to be thin/lean and somehow 20 pounds snuck up on them.
5. The avid endurance athletes who are worn out from all their training and still cannot get rid of their belly fat.
6. The yo-yo dieter whose string finally broke.

I am using your fat as my primary example point to emphasize the problems with the modern dietary and exercise programs out there. I could have used your awful fatigue, your terrible sex life, your insulin resistance, your brain fog, your high cholesterol, your depression and anxiety, your sleep issues, your blood pressure, or one of many other objective and subjective concerns to emphasize the same fallacy of modern health programs. I chose your fat because that is what most people pay attention to. Who cares what your cholesterol level or blood pressure is if you look good, right? Fat is an indicator of issues with your body. Fat obviously appears to change when you take on an extreme exercise and/or diet program, so it is a simple way to show you something is up when you do a modern exercise or diet program.

Maybe you're one of the rare ones and you quit doing the program and maintained your "new" physique for a time. How about six months later? How about a year? Two years? That's what I thought. Your fatness came back, or did it ever really leave at all? That could be argued via semantics, quantum physics, metaphysics, or pure mysticism—either way, I am not here to argue that point. I am here to help you fix what's been broken by the ridiculousness of modern, popular dieting, especially for those going through the physique-obtaining diets as professed by popular imagery and personal trainers, and the diets offered by weight loss clinics under medical supervision.

## Categories of Physique Obtaining Programs

There are many different weight loss or physique obtaining programs, diets, exercise plans, supplements, even drugs out there for people to try. I would argue they could all be classified into two distinct and separate categories, with certain bullet points being met under each heading. (See Table I)

The less than 1% of programs that don't fit this category, semantically speaking, are not diets at all. They are lifestyles. These actually work, but our "I want it **NOW**" culture refuses to see that. Unless, of course, you are at the end of your rope with your body and you realize you need to heal and repair. That is why you picked up this book, right?

| TABLE I | Modern Fat to Fit to Fat Program | Lifestyle Program |
|---|---|---|
| Length of program | 12 weeks on average | Forever |
| Goals | Short Term | Long Term |
| Food types | Restricted | Open |
| Calories | Restricted | More variability |
| Freedom to cheat | None | Available |
| Supplements | Generalized for everyone but specific to the short-term goal | Specific to the individual |
| Exercise | Excessive | Minimal |
| Stress on Body | Excessive | Minimal |
| Macronutrients | Restricted or lop-sided | Balanced to the individual |
| Drugs | Encouraged | Minimized if not removed |
| Perspective | Restricted to physical appearance | Focused on balance of mind, body, and spirit |

## How Often Do Modern Diet and Exercise Plans Work?

Studies show that only 2 to 3 percent of people who lose weight can maintain the loss for any length of time. That is dismal, at best. Talk about poor job satisfaction if you are a diet counselor, nutritionist, personal trainer, or even a doctor in the field.

For the physique world (bodybuilders, fitness girls, physique contestants, etc.), I think the percentage of those able to maintain their hard worked for body is much greater. Going through my notes and charts on thousands of patients over many years, my guess it is closer to 10–20% in the first year but then plummets to 5–8% in the fifth year.

The fact is if you go on any sort of current diet and exercise program, you eventually must stop it. Personal or forceful choice, or out of pure boredom or frustration, you must stop it. It causes relationship issues, you have a mental breakdown (or your loved ones have a mental breakdown from your choices), or just plain fatigue.

## The After Picture

In our society, we are all about the After Picture. It's all that matters. The before picture may get some notice and attention if it is unattractive, or downright disgusting. It is the after picture that people focus on, worship, and try to emulate.

We assume that "after" in this scenario means final or finished, but that is hardly (if ever) the case. The real after picture comes later —when the effects of the modern diet and exercise program take hold. In many instances, the real after picture puts the before picture to shame in terms of extremely grotesque, unattractive, or down right disgusting (by the fitness world's standards). The real after picture may show up months to years later. No one ever asks. If they did, I guarantee they would be shocked.

My circle and I often "tease" the after pictures, seen on the Internet or magazines as we know that it really is not the "done" picture. I had a hat that had the following embroidered on it: "***I am the after picture.***" I used to wear it to the gym. Some people would get it; others would not. It was a reference to the fact that having a good physique is a lifestyle choice, not an exercise program, not a diet, but a lifestyle. It may have been cocky to some, but it really was a testament to everything I am about to describe in this book.

I think, in reality, the before and after picture are one. I think one may be more obvious at any one time, but both are who you are. If this were not the case, the continual transformation from before to after to before, etc. would not be going on. The tens of thousands of before and after pictures should include a whole bunch of after pictures—maybe at 6 months, then yearly following? Whatever the chosen interval between pictures, they should be included from now on. That would provide an example of a program that really works. That would be impressive.

Hopefully you have a basic understanding of what you are about to review and learn from. It is not the easiest topic to understand or grasp as it is so contrary to everything you have been told before. To coin a fabulous term from the late 90s, "It is a paradigm shift."

I think the best way to get you thinking in terms of what is really going on with a modern diet and exercise program and why you gain all your weight back or can't lose weight in the first place is to show you what the problem is *not*.

Welcome to Chapter 2.

# CHAPTER 2
## Don't Blame Me!

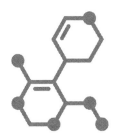

Do you have TATT syndrome: Tired All The Time? How about USTA, you know, "I USTA feel good"? Chances are if you are reading this book, you have both of these disease states. Let's get you on track to cure these terrible ailments by helping you and your body recover from the crazy "get healthy and lean" routine.

First, we need to discuss two primary things that **should not take the blame** for your failure to obtain that body you want, or your hapless attempt to feel good.

1. **Your age!**

    Repeatedly I hear in clinical practice, "Doc, it must be my age keeping me from getting leaner like I used to." I also hear, "Doctor, I am getting old so I am getting fat!" I agree; your age does matter as things change or better said, ***things get*** *harder*. Your basal metabolic rate (BMR) decreases almost linearly with age, and this appears to be related to the decrease in muscle mass as you age. Muscles consume a very large part of energy in the normal human body. Decreased muscle equals decreased metabolic rate. But this is more of a lifestyle choice than an obligation. Men and women who eat plenty of protein and utilize resistance training in their exercise regimen can control muscle mass a little better. However, this describes the avid exerciser, so why are they still having trouble obtaining or revisiting the body they want/once had? The chronic or over time effects of stress and the stress hormone cortisol play a role. Age also comes into play as the effect of time on your skin changes your appearance. I have many clients in their late forties, fi ies, and sixties with incredible bodies, but the skin hangs off a little more than it used to. Don't get loose skin and fat confused—they are different processes.

2. **You!**

   *"I let myself down"*

   Unless you are sitting around, eating whatever the next food commercial tempts you to eat, never exercising, and stressed to the hilt, it is not all your fault that you cannot obtain that body. It is very rarely a lack of motivation or effort. The fault lies in what you have been led to believe. It is the current suggested programs out there that have misled you, as well as the medical world, the food industry, and the government. Not to sound like a conspiracy theorist, but money makes people do a lot of weird things until those weird things become accepted as the norm. Give yourself a break. Let me show you how to fix it correctly. You can stop all the self-blame and depression. You can stop changing from one exercise or diet program to another, no matter how they are disguised.

The second thing we need to do is discuss the things that *get a lot of the blame* for your failure to obtain that body you want. Some of these most certainly play a role, but should not by any means get all the credit.

1. **You quit the program**

    Let's say you bought a popular DVD exercise program, literally worked your backside off, and got some good results. Then you quit the program because life happened and you lost your newfound body. You and the program disciples would tell you it is because you quit doing the DVD program. Well, let's talk quickly about why you quit doing it: You're bored, you hurt, you're hungry, you're fatigued, you're worn-out, you're moody, your kids don't like you, your husband thinks your menstrual cycle is non-stop, and your dog runs away from you when you try to pet it. This is what happens with most diet and exercise programs. Your body and mind cannot keep up the pace and naturally you start to break down. Quitting this program is probably the best thing you could do for you and your loved ones.

2. **You do not change up your program enough**

    There are books written on this one. They profess that you should…no…you *must* change your workout routine or your body gets used to the exercises and you burn fewer calories. I disagree. While changing things up is a good idea for your brain (I like saying, "Monogamy is for marriage, not the gym."), it's the intensity that burns calories no matter what you do. You could argue that the same routine brings on boredom and, therefore, decreases intensity—I agree. But back to calories—you gained your weight back not because your exercise and/or diet program got boring. It was because your exercise and/or diet program screwed up your hormones and now you're in a vicious spiral to failure, no matter what exercises you choose to do or how much you restrict your caloric intake.

3. **You are rewarding yourself incorrectly**

    You're training hard, eating little, eating specific and very limited to the suggested plan of the exercise and diet program, so you deserve to go out Friday night with the boys, have a few drinks and a pizza. Well, now this has caught up with you and you are fat again. Nope. Wrong. This is very good for mind, body, and spirit in real life (unless Friday night becomes Friday through Wednesday. Then we can throw some blame there). It's the exercise and/or diet program you are doing that is starting to change your body for the worse. Your occasional night out is of great psychologic and hormonal benefit, as you will soon discover.

4. **You're not weighing yourself often enough**

    This has been quoted time and again in journal articles, books, blogs, etc., as a factor in the failure of body morphing. It is based on the fact that regular body tracking was associated with people who were able to maintain weight loss longer than one year. The information can be found at The National Weight Control Registry (nwcr.ws) where 75% of these "successful" weight loss people weighed themselves at least once a week. Interesting finding, but correlation does not imply causation. Once you have reached the pinnacle of the diet and exercise program you are doing and real life has kicked in, you will only monitor the scale increasing, no matter how often you look at it.

5. **Other than your exercise, you do not move enough (or) you sit too much at your job (or) you need to move more**

Now with overall health, heart health, brain health, etc., yes—I agree—you need to move as much as possible. The more the better. It is called NEAT activity or Non-Exercise Activity Thermogenesis. This is your life outside of sleep and the gym. Parking farther from your destination, using the stairs rather than the escalator, tapping your foot continuously, getting up from your desk and taking a short walk every 15 min. These all use energy/calories, and therefore, if you are not doing any of them, you fail and your weight comes back. This is not true either. Yes, it is extremely good for you to move as often as possible and I highly encourage it, but since your weight and body issues are more hormonally and environmentally controlled rather than calorie-controlled, it really has little to do with fat loss or fat regain. Also, of importance to realize is the fact that if you are not a "natural exerciser" (natural athlete, loves to push yourself, likes the high of running, etc.) and you force out that exercise, you will most certainly not move the rest of the day. You will also crave sweets and other hormonally active foods to make up for that involuntary exercise. In other words, it is the overexercising and undereating that caused the weight gain in the first place!

6. **You are always missing breakfast, so you got fat again**

It could be argued that the whole breakfast thing is a product of the Kellogg Company and their target marketing years ago. The National Weight Control Registry states that 78% of its wonder people eat breakfast every day. So, is it all about breakfast? No. Wrong again. There is obviously more to it than that. I have just as many successful weight loss clients and bodybuilders who don't eat breakfast as those who do. I prescribe many programs that do not include the classical breakfast (will review in later chapters) and people do wonderfully. I am a fan of breakfast. You cannot drive your car unless you fuel it before a trip. But just adding breakfast to your morning routine will not fix your problem. Sorry.

7. **You stop paying attention to your food intake (amounts, types of food, protein, etc.)**

   This one has some truth in it, at least, but let me ask you this: **WHY** did you stop measuring, weighing, and calculating everything? Your exercise and diet program made you do it religiously, and now, due to the entirety of the program (the diet, the exercise, the supplements, the drugs, the cost, etc.), you are sick and tired of doing it. Correct? So, you get lax, but the second you see the roll return on your lower belly, you get back to it. This time it is not working! You are going to tell me (based on this incorrect assumption) that because you slacked off for a short while on your food intake you can't get your stage body back? That is what this assumption is stating, but that is far from the truth no matter how you look at it.

8. **It is because you drink coffee rather than green tea**

   Really. Seriously people. The few extra calories burned by the catechins (antioxidants found in green tea that optimize the liver and cause fat cells to release fat) do not cause enough benefits to make coffee vs. green tea even an argument! Coffee consumption has health benefits as well, unless you are drinking 10 cups a day because your ideological diet and exercise program has you so fatigued by the overexercising and undereating (*Hey…that may be the problem*. Good job, Sherlock—it **IS** the overexercising and undereating; keep reading).

9. **You went on vacation and had a huge bender (or) for you fitness/bodybuilder types: you went nuts eating everything you could get your mouth around for days or weeks following a show.**

After being on your modern diet and exercise program for any length of time, your body and brain change. Studies have shown that when you are stressed out, deprived of your favorite foods, fatigued, and lacking the "feel good" hormones in your brain, you become seriously obsessed, if not manic, when you are once again exposed, then allow yourself access to all the delectable treats you can imagine. I know bodybuilders who have put on 20+ pounds in a few days. Now most of this is water of course, but it sets the course for bad things happening. Hormonally, it can be good if you can control it (we will cover this in detail when we get into how to fix this), but in most cases control never returns. Does this cause the seemingly per-petual change in your body that is now ruined? No—it does not. It is what you did to your body *before* the binge that caused the issue; in other words, it was not the binge, but the up-to-date diet and exercise program that caused all the issues in the first place.

10. **Calories-in-to-Calories-out**

Calories-in-to-calories-out gets most of the attention. The general rule of any good exercise and/or diet program out there is based on the calorie myth. Eat less and exercise more—that is the basic tenet of any/all of the modern diet and exercise programs. Several of the falsities I spoke about above are inadvertently blaming you for eating too many calories or not exercising enough of them off. Let me spend a few paragraphs helping you see through that myth.

Before I get into my own personal revelation about the calorie myth, let me start with some basic science: When calories are restricted, an enzyme called lipoprotein lipase dramatically increases. Lipoprotein lipase is a lipogenic or fat-storing enzyme. The body senses the decreased calories and starts protecting itself by storing more fat.

Triiodthyronine or T3, the active thyroid hormone, also decreases, something we will talk about in more detail later. T3 downregulates to protect muscle but, in doing so, it also protects fat. The more calories you restrict (and the more calories you burn with exercise), the more your body increases lipoprotein lipase and decreases T3. This is one of the reasons you gain weight so quickly following a modern exercise and diet program. This enzyme and hormone take a while to adjust to the higher calorie intake of "normal eating," so the excess calories (compared to your restricted amount) are stored as fat.

On the other extreme, if calories-in-to-calories-out is true, simple math tells us that we should have many 5000-pound people in the world. If you consumed 1000 calories more than you need every day for a year (that's two "luxury" coffees a day), and did not change your exercise/activity level and, as a pound of fat is equivalent to 3500 calories, you would gain over 100 pounds a year. Do that for three years, and you are now 313 pounds heavier. Since we know this does not happen, there must be other things going on. As your caloric intake increases, your metabolic rate increases, due in part to a down regulation of lipoprotein lipase and an increase in T3. In other words, the fatter you are, the higher your metabolic rate—not the other way around! There is simply not a linear relationship between caloric intake, caloric expenditure, and your degree of fatness (or leanness).

Why are some people more apt to gain fat with increased caloric intake? Studies have shown that there is an intra-human, genetically determined, variance of fat storage (up to a ten-fold difference) in response to caloric consumption. Genetics are not the end all in this equation, however—it is a multifactorial thing including epi-genetics (there is a quick discussion on epi-genetics in the FAQ section of the book) and a hormonal phenomenon involving a large number of different hormones including insulin (discussed in the next few paragraphs) and glucagon.

# Personal Revelation into the Calorie Myth

I started helping people with their health and body goals over 30 years ago, as a personal trainer. Like all personal trainers at the time (and there were not that many of us back then!), I believed that if you were not reaching your body goals, you simply needed to eat less and exercise more. As time progressed, my education became more involved, and I began to understand the human body, human physiology, and the powerful effects of food on the body. I also began to question this universally held belief. Something was amiss, but I simply could not grasp what. All the pieces seemed to fit in the puzzle, but the picture of the puzzle did not look right. Every effort to find out what was wrong seemed to lead to another dead end.

In the 1980s and early 1990s, I worked as a nutritional consultant with several athletes who performed at all levels of competitive sports. Some of the athletes I worked with, including those on the professional level, utilized hormones to their advantage. Many of them employed anabolic androgenic steroids (AAS) to improve performance, optimize muscularity, and develop the "Adonis" physique. These steroids, or hormones, had a powerful impact on their users and, depending on many factors, improved their body composition no matter how many calories were being eaten or burned in the gym. At this point in my career, I could tell hormones (amongst other things) had a powerful effect on the body; I just could not grasp the detail yet.

When I got into medical school and started learning all about biochemistry, physiology, and the power of hormones in our bodies, I started trying some nutritional theories I had been developing on some of these same people. Rather than being so concerned about exactly how much or how little they ate, I started to develop eating plans based on the effects certain foods were having on the body. I began to realize that it was not so much the food they ate, but what their bodies were doing with that food, that really made a difference in physical attributes such as fat gain, fat loss, muscle gain, and muscle loss. This is when I originally developed the theory and practice of "Food Timing." It was becoming more apparent to me that the time certain foods were eaten throughout the day was a powerful regulator of fat loss and muscle gain. This eating style was based on the metabolic state of the body, the natural circadian rhythm of the body (or how the body's metabolic state follows the natural daily rhythm of the sun rising and setting), and when the body was stressed, such as during vigorous exercise. "Food Timing" became a powerful way of eating that has helped tens of thousands of people optimize their physiques (i.e., lose fat and gain muscle). The importance of hormones and body composition, rather than counting calories-in and calories-out, was becoming apparent.

In early 1997, while having dinner with a top-level athlete who was a client of mine, my then-theory was confirmed. While eating at a restaurant with this very large, muscular gentleman and his girlfriend, he became noticeably ill right before my eyes. For some reason our food was delayed, and he seemed to take notice more than the rest of us. He started sweating profusely, his face turned white, and his speech started to slur. He got up out of his chair and stumbled outside, falling to the sidewalk in front of the restaurant. I started an emergency evaluation of my large friend.

First, I made sure he had an airway open and that he was breathing. His breathing was shallow and very rapid, and his pulse was extremely fast. His skin was hot, wet, and clammy. I asked the maître d' to help us and then quickly turned to his girlfriend. I asked her if he had been doing anything different, unusual, or out of the ordinary that she could think of. In the back of my mind, I was concerned about drug use. He was an admitted anabolic androgenic steroid user and once any drug such as that is utilized, there seems to be no limit to what other drugs these good people may use to optimize their performance and physique. His girlfriend stated that she had seen him inject something in his belly before each meal over the last month or two.

It hit me like a ton of bricks. I had been hearing rumors of this practice during the World Games, as well as during the Olympics. My thoughts went immediately to the drug insulin. My nondiabetic, normal pancreatic functioning friend was utilizing insulin as an anabolic (muscle building) aid. I felt sure I had made the right diagnosis and, therefore, knew what intervention needed to be made. I had the maître d' grab some bags of sugar and a glass of water for me. I put the sugar in my hand and mixed some water with it, pried his mouth open, and started rubbing the sugar water under his tongue and around his gums and lips.

He started responding rather quickly and, within a matter of minutes, he could drink the last of the sugar water.

It was rather fascinating. A drug utilized by diabetics to control blood sugar was being used by a non-diabetic to enhance muscular growth.

This practice was literally unheard of in the medical world and, following this little event, I wrote the first reported case study in medical literature about utilizing a blood sugar hormone as an anabolic aid. If you are interested in reading it, here is the reference:

## Insulin as an AnabolicAid?The Physician and Sports Medicine:Vol 25, No.10; October 1997, Dr.Warren Willey

When my athletic friend regained his composure and thought process, I asked him the exact nature of his insulin use. He and most others in his sport had been utilizing insulin over the preceding year as an anabolic aid. It was well known by this subculture of athletes that insulin is probably the most powerful growth-promoting hormone in the body. Utilizing insulin like this is, of course, very dangerous and deadly. I have seen a few case reports of athletes dying from this practice since I first reported it. But the fact was my client's experience made that puzzle I described earlier become crystal clear. The pieces of the puzzle fit together perfectly, and the picture created was a beautiful composition of colors and a burst of understanding. A big part of the secret to weight gain, weight loss, muscle gain, and fat loss is hormones.

Bariatric or obesity surgery has been used in the calories-in-to-calories-out theory for some time. The belief is that, if one can change how many calories are absorbed into the body by changing the normal anatomy (such as limiting the size of the stomach or limiting areas of absorption), then the patient will lose weight. While this is true to a point, bariatric surgery changes hormones and changes the gut bacteria. Before the surgery, the patient will meet with a nonsurgical, obesity medicine specialist, who will stop most, if not all, medications. This includes blood pressure medication, cholesterol medication, diabetic medication, and any other medication or chronic disease drugs. We do this because the hormonal and gut bacteria change associated with this surgery is so drastic these medications are no longer needed after the surgery! If it was purely a calorie absorption issue, we would require these medications until the weight was lost, which in some cases may take months. What happens after surgery? The surgery changes hormones and gut bacteria and these are helping to dictate weight loss.

Bariatric surgeons have recognized the importance of hormones and other metabolic processes in weight loss. So much so, that they changed the name of their organization to reflect this. They went from The American Society of Bariatric Surgery, to The American Society for *Metabolic* and Bariatric Surgery.

If you have God-given, functional anatomy removed by a surgeon, and if weight loss was simply a caloric issue, one would expect it would be impossible to regain weight following surgery. Right? But many of us know someone who has gained weight back following bariatric surgery. How did they gain the weight back? Their environment or lifestyle did not change with the surgery.

Let me tell you how to "cure" bariatric surgery, once again, showing it is not a calorie issue but a hormonal, psychiatric, toxin, environmental issue.

The story of this particular cure came from a post-bariatric surgical patient, via a fellow obesity medicine specialist, who then shared the story at the American Society of Bariatric Medicine conference I was a guest lecturer for. This sweet lady admits to becoming as large as possible to keep people away from her following a very traumatic childhood experience. She was convinced by doctors to have the surgery to improve her health. After the surgery, she lost hundreds of pounds. She was lean and attractive, and this gave her great anxiety and fear, as memories and trepidation returned from her childhood experiences So, she cured her bariatric surgery. She drank Karo Syrup. For those of you who do not know, Karo Syrup is pure corn syrup—a 100% hormone-stimulating drug and very toxic in and of itself. In a very short period, she gained back the weight she had lost, and then some. It is important to understand that it would be virtually impossible to drink enough calories in Karo Syrup to gain that much weight (making it a non-calorie issue). But if you change the beneficial hormonal response and expose the body to a bad toxin, then yes, you can cure bariatric surgery and gain back the weight.

Calories-in-to-calories-out dominated both the medical and lay literature. As I travel a lot, speaking and going to medical conferences, I have had the opportunity to talk with some of the world's best in the weight loss field. They too hint that something else is going on besides calories-in-to-calories-out but when pressed for details, they always came back to the comfort of the calorie equation. It appears that when these incredibly smart individuals questioned the role of calories, as I have been doing, they threw up their hands and simply accepted it. This acceptance is based solely on the fact that it had been accepted by those who had come before them and there was no alternative.

I could go on, but I think you get the point. Common misconceptions taken as scientific fact are fallacies and products of marketing. Yes, these factors may play a role in your inability to lose fat, but not one or even two of them, or all of them for that matter made it impossible for you to get the physique you want. There is something else going on here, and you know it!

## Fat Is Adaptive

Before we dive in, I think there is something I should let you in on. It took me a long time to figure this out, but now that I see it, it makes total sense. I hope it opens your eyes as well.

We are in a society that continually harps and complains about fat. Fat is criminalized both in our mouths and on our bodies. Disease states such as cancer and heart disease are directly linked to it. *Prejudice* and meanness abound toward people with any sort of fat on them. We have grown up thinking that fat is the product of gluttony and sloth. You are fat because you eat too much and don't move enough. This fallacy is what gives modern exercise and diet programs their energy and popularity. If this absurdity were true, then the only way to conquer it would be to eat less (diet) and move more (exercise). Yes—that does work in the short run, but anyone who has done it is also one who has failed at it. Even if it takes a few years, failure is inevitable. I will cover this more in the book as we go along, but my point in this section is for you to consider this: We have come to believe that fat is *maladaptive*. You have fat because of a problem with your movement and eating.

## I absolutely disagree with that. Fat is *not* maladaptive.
## *Fat is adaptive.*

The definition of adaptation in Merriam-Webster's Dictionary is *modification of an organism or its parts that makes it more fit for existence under the conditions of its environment.* In other words, it is our environment, including toxins, stress, hormonal changes, lack of sleep, etc., that the body adapts to via storing fat.

Toxins for example. Where do you think your body stores toxins when you are exposed to them? It's not in your heart or brain, as the toxins would kill you. The majority of toxins you are exposed to are stored in your fat. It's not reported too often, but a large percentage of people gain their weight back or die after bariatric surgery, after they have lost the fat. Why? The fat released toxins with the weight loss and the other organs cannot take them. If those toxins do not kill you, your body will store fat again to protect you. We are surrounded by toxins. In the plastics you microwave your food in to your fast food meal that has a shelf life a lot longer than you do, or the fumes from the semi-truck in front of you as you sit in hours of traffic getting to and from work each day, to the weed killer you spray in your child's sandbox...the list goes on. Toxins are everywhere and unless you have a stellar clearance system (which some people do via their livers, kidneys, sweat in the gym, etc.), your body protects you by adapting to the environmental exposures/toxins and storing fat to keep those chemicals away from vital organs.

Another example as to why fat is adaptive is the fact that, fat itself is a vital organ. Our bodies will do anything/everything to protect it. It is a producer of some of the most important hormones in the body, mother hormones, in my opinion, as they have the ability to control or override many other hormones. This is one of the reasons someone could have a dysfunctional thyroid or sex hormones, despite normal lab results. Two of these fat produced hormones, leptin and adiponectin, are powerhouses in the body. Adiponectin helps rid the body of toxins and even helps remove bad visceral fat (fat around the organs in your gut) from your body.

Fat accumulates in a protective manner due to hormonal changes, lack of sleep, and stress including mental, physical, and emotional pressures. Fat is your body's adaptation to your environment! It is not just the result of laziness and bad eating.

When you do go full out on the exercise and eating correctly, that is, a contemporary exercise and diet program, your body adapts to the low calories and high exercise amounts by slowing things down—the metabolic damage you hear about. Fat accumulation increases in response to this "metabolic damage." In other words—fat is adaptive.

Hopefully, that raised some eyebrows out there because once you grasp this concept, you will see the fallacy of a currently suggested diet and exercise program. Popular programs have you eat very little and exercise very a lot (I know the English is off there, but I liked the sound of it). You change in size or get leaner, but if your environment has not changed, your fat will come back with a vengeance to protect you. Your body, from the neck down, does not care what you look like. Its job is to protect and support you from the neck up! If that means building more and more fat to do it, it will do just that. No questions asked; it does not care if you like it or not. It is doing its job. Period.

To change your fat, you must change your environment. To change your environment, you must understand what the modern diet and exercise recommendations are doing to you. You must then recognize how to fix it. The fix part is a little more complicated, but I think this book will give you some direction or, at the very least, point you in the right direction to get some help fixing it.

To get you started, I am providing you with some real-life case studies of actual people who did aggressive diet and exercise programs and their journeys to being healed.

# CHAPTER 3
## Case Studies of People Just Like You

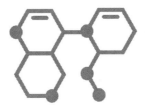

I see the fallacy of modern diet and exercise programs daily in my practice. Somedays, it is all I see. My practice is admittedly determined to see this problem. I think a lot of people who come to my office with other complaints such as severe fatigue, brain fog, lack of sex drive, etc., have this issue without realizing it.

I am using this chapter to let you visit and hear the stories of a few of my patients that I think you are likely to relate to. But before I get into the detailed case studies of these fine people, let me share with you a couple of emails I got today while writing this chapter. I get emails like this daily. I see a lot of people with these concerns, but I get even more emails than I do patients with this and similar concerns. The first email was titled:

***Female 54 and Frustrated***

Dr. Willey: Can you tell me why 1 year ago I had lost 40 pounds taking some medications *(the list has been removed)*

---------5 mg a day

---------50 mg

---------15 mg

I worked with a trainer

Got to goal weight 149. Body fat 24%

Now 1 year later I'm back up to 166 on no medication and working with a trainer again.

Lifting 6 days a week plus 1 or 2 spinning classes for an hour plus

30 min cardio the 4 or 5 other days a week.

What gives? Plus 1200–1300 calories a day!!!

How do I get an appointment with you?

The second email was from a personal trainer on behalf of her client (who happened to be a patient of mine as well) titled:

*Need Help…*

Hi Dr Willey,
This is xxxxx from xxxxx Athletic Club. I am working with xxxxx. She recently met with you and said she gave you permission to speak with me about her medical history.

She has struggled with weight loss for a long time. She is getting really frustrated. Did her blood tests show anything significant? Here is where I am stuck…She does lose weight, but seems to just go back and forth between 158 and 144. But, when she gets back up to her high point, she is able to drop back down but never below 144, so I know that she isn't broken!

She lifts weights 6 days per week. From what she logs, her diet is on point. She is currently consuming 1400 cals which I actually think is low for her. (99 carbs with 25 fiber, less than 39 sugar, 44 fat, 143 protein). I hate to drop her down to 1200, but I am wondering if a temporary drop doing some cycling with her calories would help. We have done some carb cycling also. We have changed her macros around a few times to see if we can find her sweet spot.

This is her workout routine. She also either does ballet, plays tennis or bowls 4 nights a week. She is on a mid-rep weights routine, and this is what her schedule looks like:

Monday: Warm up 5 min, Weights for 45, HIIT on treadmill for 25

Tuesday: Warm up 10 min, Weights for 60, Stretch 10

Wednesday: Warm up 5 min, Weights for 30, Steady state on stepper for 45

Thursday: Warm up 10 min, Weights for 60 min, Stretch 10

Friday: Warm up 5 min, Weights for 30, Steady state on treadmill for 45

Saturday: Warm up 5 min, Weights for 1.5, 30 min HIIT on stepper/bike

My next step is to flip her cardio and her weights to see if putting more of a focus on cardio will help. She does gain lean mass easy, so I don't think this would hurt.

Any advice would help!

Thanks,

xxxxxx

Both emails exemplify what I do day in and day out. The first young lady is suffering from the results of a personal trainer program a year later, and the young lady described in the second email is currently undergoing a modern high exercise, low calorie program and is extremely frustrated as to why she is not changing despite the obvious work and effort she is putting forth. These are real problems and real concerns. As you can read in the emails, both of these people are desperate for a solution to their body concerns and want answers as to why—everything they have been taught or have been doing—is not working or does not work in the long run. Frustration does not run much higher.

Below are real people with real stories. The ex-college athlete wrote her story herself. She did a much better job telling it than I would, as it includes real life details and stresses that contributed to her problem. My medical assistant, Lisa, wrote about the most common patient I (we) see in my medical practice as we have become somewhat sought out for this condition. The other five people are actual clients of mine who suffered greatly until they listened to me (their words, not mine).

## The Once-Upon-a-Time Bodybuilder

Jon was like a lot of recently divorced men of his age. Late-thirties, now single, and back on the dating scene. It was a rough divorce and his comfort food acted as his only antidepressant/anti-anxiety medication. Great medicine for the time being, but it had terrible side effects for a man who wanted to start dating again—he got fat. He had always been in good shape, exercising most days of the week before the divorce, but he let himself go this time. He knew that if he was going to have any luck with the cute girls at the gym or his office, he had to look amazing. He was and always had been a goal-driven person, so he set his sights on a bodybuilding show exactly one year from the time he decided to get back into shape. Why not? He had always toyed with the idea, but the commitment was too great when he had a family. He was going to transform his life and go for it!

He changed his comfort drugs from cookies and ice cream (or pizza and beer on the weekends) to time in the gym. He got up earlier each day to prepare his food. He watched and read fitness blogs and YouTube videos every break he had, to learn as much as he could about bodybuilding. He scanned Bodybuilding.com for everything he could read on getting in contest shape. As a now single guy, he had lots of time for the gym, working out two or three hours most days of the week. He made some progress, and was feeling good, but that six pack was still hiding under a layer of fat and he could not get his legs to respond and grow, no matter what workout he tried or saw on YouTube. Frustrated, he started asking around the gym as to what to do and who would be the person to help him. Universally, everyone he spoke to said to talk to Craig.

Craig was a personal trainer and worked in a few of the gyms in town. He was considered the best personal trainer in the area for bodybuilding and physique shows, as all of his clients not only got into show shape, but many of them placed very well in the competitions. Craig was the guy to go to, so Jon did just that—he made a consult appointment with Craig.

Craig himself was the Adonis figure. About six foot tall, 225 pounds, lean, and muscular, he had won many shows over the years. He was the perfect guy for Jon to have train him, as he not only looked like how Jon wanted to look, but had helped many people get to where Jon wanted to be. *Perfect*, Jon thought to himself. *I don't care what this guy charges, I am going for it.* Charge him he did, but for a good reason, so said Craig: "I am the best and I will get you where you want to be." Jon only hesitated for a moment thinking to himself about the cost of the divorce and alimony, money for the kids, etc. *Nope*—he said to himself, *it's worth it because it is what I want.*

Craig started training Jon right away. They met three times a week for absolutely killer workouts (Jon admitted to me he often threw up afterward and felt dizzy for hours following) and on days Craig did not train him, he had a very strict routine to follow. "No questions asked," said Craig. "If you want to be in a show, you *must* do what I say." Jon trained as hard as he could when Craig was not there, as he did not want to fail or disappoint him.

Craig also wrote his diet. It came on a computer printed page, a word document, and seemed almost rote, as if it had been used before, but Jon did not care. This was it! This was what he was looking for. He knew for sure he was going to get there. The diet was hard and expensive. Twelve egg whites with one cup of steel cut oats for breakfast every day. A protein shake for snack at 10:00 a.m., followed by 10 ounces of chicken, and ½ cup of brown rice for lunch. For the afternoon snack, it was another protein drink/shake and 5 hardboiled egg whites. Dinner was 8 ounces of fish or game meat cooked in olive oil, 5 broccoli spears, ½ of an avocado, and salad if he was still hungry. Plain salad, no dressing or additives. If he was hungry at night, he could have another protein shake again, but 1/3 the size of the protein shake he had in the afternoon. Craig emphasized that it was best if he did not use it and he should just go to bed if he was starving.

Craig had a list of supplements that also came on a preprinted, wrinkled word document—a pre-workout powder that always made Jon feel nauseous, but he had energy when he trained (then crashed later!) It listed a funny-named supplement called Trenavar (which he later found out was a popular prohormone), creatine monohydrate twice a day, and some Branch Chain Amino Acids (BCAA), and a few others that he could not remember all the names for.

Jon ate just as he was told, day in and day out, right off the menu and supplement list. Monotony and boredom did not bother him as he was going to succeed. Why not? Craig looked the part, and obviously knew what he was doing, so Jon ate the same thing every day, seven days a week, without fail. "No questions asked," said Craig, so Jon did not ask them.

Jon leaned up some more and was progressing great until he hit a wall. The wall was not obvious in the gym. The pre-workout supplement allowed him to push through anything, including being fatigued and nauseous, but he still had this roll of fat on his lower belly. His legs improved, but looked nothing like Craig's or anyone's on Bodybuilding.com's front page. Jon was getting frustrated, but kept pushing.

Eventually, Jon's personal life started to suffer. His friends and support group that had helped him through his divorce stopped asking him to go out on the weekends because he always turned them down so he could stick to his diet. He started waking up at night between 1:00 and 3:00 a.m. on a regular basis and was lacking sleep. His moods changed, he was always on edge, and barked at his co-workers, feeling terrible afterward. It was as if he knew he was being an ass, but could not control it. When he was not exercising, he felt like crap. He was tired, mentally drained, emotional, lacking motivation for anything but the gym. But no matter, he had a goal, and he was going to continue pursuing it, no matter what the consequences.

That darn belly fat! Jon asked Craig about it and his legs—why were they not improving with the amount of effort he was putting in? He confronted Craig on it. How could anyone work so hard and still have skinny legs and belly fat? At this point, Jon, while telling me the whole story, said Craig's face changed. His eyes got narrow and his brow dropped, and Craig asked him, "Are you ready to go to the next level?"

Of course, Jon was ready for the next level. How could one not be after the effort he was putting in? Craig asked, "Are you willing to take it there?" Jon of course answered YES, as his entire life had changed to get as far as he had. "What do I have to do?" asked Jon.

Craig pulled two bottles of pills from his gym bag and said, "These are not cheap, but will get you there." The bottles were not labeled, as if a prescription bottle for Amoxicillin had the label pulled off.

"Take one of these three times a day and take two of these twice a day," Craig said. Jon did not hesitate. If these were going to help him reach his goal, so be it! Jon only hesitated for a minute to ask what they were, but admittedly, never asked anything beyond that.

"The one you take two of twice a day is called Anavar, the one you take one of three times a day is called Clenbuterol. The Clenbuterol may cause your heart to race, but don't worry about that. It's normal."

Craig then pulled out a small dark bottle of liquid with a home computer printed label. "This is Testosterone. You need a boost and this will help. Take 2 cc (mL) every 4 days; here are some syringes and needles." Craig then demonstrated how to inject himself with the drug. "It may hurt a little but don't worry about that—it's worth it!" Jon did not hesitate. If his goal was to be reached, he would do it. After all, Craig obviously knew what he was doing. Look at him.

Jon spent the money and started taking the pills and injections just as Craig had suggested. His heart did race, almost to the point of making him think it was going to bounce right out of his chest! He thought about going to his doctor, but he felt dirty for taking the medication and did not want to be judged. His butt hurt for days following the injections, but he did not care. His goal was to be reached!

Over the next few weeks, Jon's legs started to respond to the heavy, almost debilitating, squats. His belly fat started to go away. *A six pack—NO, maybe an eight pack! I knew it was there!* thought Jon excitedly.

Jon followed this course for the next few months and really started to look like a bodybuilder. He started standing in front of his bathroom mirror comparing himself to guys he saw on YouTube and Bodybuilding.com. *I can do this! I am there!* he would say to himself.

He stuck to the diet, trained hard, took the drugs as suggested, and looked the role. He felt girls in the gym and at work were paying attention to him. *This is great*, he would say to himself. In retrospect, he realized he was in a different world. Not a real world, but certainly a different world. His work and personal life were in shambles, but no matter—he was after a goal!

Jon did the contest exactly one year after he set the goal. He did well, placing third in the over 35 division of an NPC (National Physique Committee) bodybuilding show.

He was on cloud 9. Nothing could stop him now. He asked Craig what to do after the show. Craig told him, "Have fun for a few days with eating and drinking beer with your buddies, but let's get back to the gym after you take off a couple of weeks."

Jon did just that. He ate, and ate, and ate—then he drank beer like it was water. *I deserve this*, he would say to himself. *I worked hard and this is my reward!*

His body seemed to be holding the shape it was in, even with the food and beer. "Wow! I can always look like this, no matter what I do!"

Jon decided he could go a little longer without contacting Craig. He was looking amazing. He actually looked better a few days after the show than he had on stage! He did not need help now—he had made it and all was good!

Over the next few weeks, Jon, feeling comfortable in his new body still exercised and did his best to eat right, but he had the occasional "cheat night," as he deserved it.

He stopped all the drugs and supplements Craig had suggested because for one it cost a lot of money and, two, he did not need them now! He was finally where he wanted to be. He did notice, as now he was full speed on the dating scene with the cute girls from the gym AND work that his sexual function started to decline. He could no longer maintain an erection like he used to. It started to bother him (and the girls he was with), but he felt it was just stress from work and it would be fine.

Until that dreadful day, Jon woke up and that roll of belly fat was back. *What!* he said to himself. *Where did that come from?* Sexual function continued to decline to the point he stopped going out with the cute girls from the gym. Nothing was working. He could not even get an erection now. He started getting tired and his job performance started to decline. *I just have to get back to the gym and train harder*, he thought. So he did. It only seemed to make matters worse.

He contacted Craig—"Let's get back on schedule, but I don't want to do any of the drugs I was doing." Craig was fine with that, but warned him it would be harder. Jon worked out to the point of being sick like he had getting ready for the show. He ate perfectly, ignoring his friends who were excited to have him back, to the point they quickly gave up on him again. He was doing everything right, but his legs shrank and his belly kept getting fatter, no matter what he did. His sleep went to hell, his moods became uncontrollable, and he eventually got back to the look and weight he had started from. He was at the end of his rope. He even admitted to me that he had contemplated suicide, as he was so depressed.

That's when a friend, who stuck with him even though he was an ass, told him to come see me. "I know this doctor who deals with this kind of stuff," he was told. Jon made an appointment and came and saw me.

When we first met, he acted tough, as if he knew it all. Five minutes into his story, I told him I knew the rest of it, and the tough guy he was broke down in tears.

I spent the next hour explaining what had happened to his body: the Fat to Fit program, including the supplements and the drugs. He would not have a chance unless we fixed the underlying problem that the Fat to Fit program had caused. That problem included his mind, his emotions, his hormones, his body. I asked him if he was ready to venture into the unknown and trust me, no matter how long it took. Would he be willing to spend some money for testing to figure it out as it was worth it (he had kids; what price could you put on them needing their father??). Besides, it was not nearly the cost of his trainer, the status quo supplements, and the drugs.

He agreed and we got to work. We tested his stress level with a cortisol test. We checked his gut health after the diet, the drugs, and the high cortisol/stress levels. We checked all his hormones at the right time of day and controlling for all variables. I had my dietitian write an eating plan for him that worked for his schedule and was personalized for him, so the cookies and ice cream were not needed anymore. I started him on a personalized supplement schedule based on his labs, and an easy exercise program twice a week with walking on days not in the gym. I adjusted his hormones with supplements and a few prescriptions, short term, to help him get back on track.

The biggest challenge was his patience and self-esteem. Going from that kind of body to what he had now was very hard, as it would be for anyone. To his credit, he hung in there for the long haul. It helped that we balanced his stress hormone, cortisol, and brain hormones concurrently, followed in short order by fixing his gut (this order is very important, as you will see later on). This allowed him to feel better, sleep better, and perform better at work, even without the Adonis physique he had become accustomed to.

Over time, his body started to change. He started to lean up again without the vigorous exercise and without the drugs or suggested bodybuilding supplements or terribly restrictive diet. He started feeling good, and his body followed in long order (vs. short order, as most would hope).

It took two years for Jon to get back to his goal. *His new goal, that is.* He was lean, 12% body fat, not 6% body fat like he was at the bodybuilding show. He felt good, had a good and steady relationship with a nice girl from work—not someone who was just after his body. He was doing great at work, his kids liked him, and he even developed a working relationship with his ex-wife—something important to him and his kids.

It was not easy, and taking two years vs. the Fat to Fit program that had gotten him there in a few months was hard, but he did it. And now he will maintain it for life. Is that not what we are all after?

## **The Fitness Girl**

Jane was a wonderful, hardworking, successful 42-year-old girl who had a dream. She wanted to do a fitness show. She was a regular exerciser, she ate well, according to her (limited meat, a lot of vegetables and fruit, and avoided fast food and pop), she practiced meditation and had a good prayer life to keep her stress down, and had a great family, with a supportive husband and wonderful kids.

She was a self-admitted fat kid and the teasing from others and the torture she put on herself because of it have never left her. She looked good and she knew it. Her husband explicitly stated it, her friends all admitted jealousy, asking how she could do it, and young men in the gym reminded her of it, as they often interrupted her workouts to hit on her!

But she wanted to take it to the next level. She wanted to beat her childhood fears and get on stage in front of many people, in less cotton than a Q-tip, and show her body. She was going to do a fitness show. She had the personality to do it, the body to do it, and the support to do it. Stand back! She was on a mission!

So, she started doing it. She took it to the next level, hiring a personal trainer from her area, a well-known fitness showgirl who had won multiple contests, including on a national level, and started a vigorous program.

She started training six days a week, changed her diet to a low carb, low calorie eating plan that left her quite hungry most of the day, but no matter—she had the audacity to do it. Nothing was going to stop her. Her trainer warned her of the hunger and suggested she do one of two things: Take a supplement to help limit her hunger or go to her doctor and get some Phentermine to help control it. She was on the straight and narrow, so she went to her doctor and got a prescription of the appetite control drug, Phentermine. This really helped and she felt great and thought to herself, *This is easy! I should have done this a long time ago.*

She was working hard and progressing fine, but it was trying. Her husband loved she was doing it, but openly admitted to her that he missed their date nights. They used to go out to dinner once a week or to a movie and eat popcorn until they got sick. This was no longer an option, as she was on a mission. Her kids missed their weekends, as they used to do fun stuff like bowling, going to the trampoline house, going out for pizza, etc. She no longer did that as she had a goal to obtain. You can't go bowling, as throwing that ball could hurt your biceps and forearm. You cannot go to the trampoline house and risk injury to your back, and you certainly cannot go to Pizza Hut, as that was not on the eating plan—even if you just ate from the salad bar, the chemicals they use to keep the salad looking "fresh" would be devastating to the body.

It was a sacrifice, but she was willing to make it. Her family was understanding, as far as she knew, and she kept on her goal.

She progressed well. Her trainer was excited, as it was obvious she was a natural and even caught on to the posing and positioning needed to get on stage.

She kept working out, training hard, eating right, and stayed on the medication to help with the hunger. Everything was going great. Her trainer could not have been happier, as someone like this was a notch in her gun.

As she approached the show, about three weeks out, her trainer really came to grips with her potential. This lady could be something else. Her trainer approached her and wanted to make sure she really dialed it in for the stage. "Let's take you to 800 calories a day just to make sure you lean up enough for the show." Jane agreed even through it frightened her a little. 800 calories a day? That's not much, but her trainer had won national shows; she must know what she is doing.

Her trainer also suggested some Clenbuterol and Anavar, but she was a purist so she refused, dropped her calories to 800 a day, and kept training hard.

Contest time finally was here. She felt great. Her family was proud of her. Her friends were so jealous they could not stand it, but supported her as she had done it. As a matter of fact, at the show over fifty people came to cheer her on.

She did rather well. As a matter of fact, she won her height class and it was a close call for the overall show title. She kicked butt and took names. She was unstoppable. She was so proud. Her family and friends praised her, she was on cloud 9, and was convinced she had found her new passion.

Following the show, being an attentive and wise woman, she did not binge or overeat. She had a nice meal with her family and friends following the show, but got right back on her diet and eating plan afterward. Reverse Dieting her trainer called it. The Monday following the Saturday show, she was right back to it. The only difference being, she increased her calories to 1300 a day. How could that hurt her? Although 1300 calories were still very low for her body, it should allow her to maintain "the look."

She cut back on her workouts as well. As her family put up with exercising six days a week while she got ready for the show, she cut back to five days a week to be with them on Saturday, and still easily maintain her physique. That was still more than twice what her friends would do. It should be easy to maintain her new, contest winning body and continue with life as it was before she got ready for the show. Right?

Reality hit her about three weeks after the show. She started gaining weight. She told me in our first consult, she was "gaining weight like crazy." Her belly, that she never had a problem with, started getting fat on it. Her thighs started to thicken, no matter how many lunges she did. She became emotional. Her menstrual cycle, which had stopped a few months back with her extreme dieting, started again, but this time with such a terrible premenstrual syndrome that even her loving husband wanted nothing to do with her for two weeks of the month. She lost all sex drive, and her sexual function deteriorated to the point she never wanted to have sex, making her husband even more concerned about her. Her kids started fearing her, as she became snappy and mean. This was really bothering her as she knew there was no reason to be upset. She would blow up at the simplest stuff, yell and scream at her kids and husband, and then feel so terrible that she spun even farther down into her depression.

She eventually gained 15–20 pounds more than she had had on her delicate frame before the contest. She dealt with constant muscle soreness that made it difficult even to get out of bed in the morning. She was at her wits' end, tired, angry, and needing help. She had non-stop abdominal pain and loose stools. She said she had to plan her activity around the closest bathroom, as the diarrhea got so bad. She was in shambles and needed help.

She went to her primary care doctor who made several referrals including to a gastroenterologist to get an endoscopy and colonoscopy for her belly symptoms. All the workups and money spent, not to mention the invasive procedures, provided her with no understanding or relief. It was time for her to seek out different help.

That's where I came in. She had read a few of my books years before, and was hopeful that I might have some insight as to her problem. Our first meeting was tearful and difficult for her. She was in pain and broke down a couple of times as I was listening to her story. After I got the whole story, I told her I had heard it before. She looked at me with disbelief. She was convinced there was a severe medical issue going on, never once thinking it could be a common phenomenon, especially with people who had competed in a physique show. How could something so healthy, turn out to be so bad?

I spent a lot of time describing the physiology behind what her body, mind, and emotions were going through. The hormones, the neurotransmitters, the stress her Fat to Fit program put on her, and the resulting consequences. "Isn't this common knowledge with that crowd?" she asked. "Why didn't my trainer tell me this could/would happen?" I helped her understand that the process/program has been done for so long it is practically gospel. No one ever thought there might be a fallacy with the technique, as the common thinking is, *If you fail it is YOUR fault, not the system's.*

Once she grasped the concept (as I said, she was a very smart woman), it hit her like a ton of bricks. The stress of the program (or if we are talking hormones: the continuous elevation of cortisol and extremely low leptin levels), actually caused the problem. Her body fought what she did to it while getting ready for the show, but it took time to respond and fight back. The Fat to Fit program **CAUSED** the problem. Once the body had time to respond and defend itself from the stress of the program, it did.

I used the sport of boxing as an example. I saw a YouTube video of a fighter who was beating his opponent very easily. He got really cocky and started parading around the ring to show his superiority. In doing so, he let his competitor rest and gain some strength. When they got back to the punches, his once weaker opponent was now ready to fight, and due to his cockiness and not paying attention, he got his backside kicked.

We ran the standard set of labs for Jane, as she wanted to be cost-conscious. She had spent a lot of money getting ready for the show, but wanted to be frugal now (author's comment: This has always stumped me—spend ungodly amounts of cash on a show or program, or trainer, but be cheap when you are sick and want to feel better). We ran a thyroid panel, sex hormones at the right time of month, chemistries—the works.

All were within normal limits.

This really freaked Jane out. "How could everything be normal when I feel like this? I am getting fat; I have become an emotional wreck!! I am falling apart and my labs are normal?" I explained to Jane that this is why this condition is missed by so many doctors and standard medical practices. Unless you understand the pathophysiology behind it and look in the right places, there is very little objective data to go on. In western medicine, when the objective data is sparse, it becomes a problem with your head. The most common medication prescribed by the average doctor who hears this story? Antidepressants. Occasionally antipsychotics, as the victims present with such distress, doctors think they are crazy!

As I told her, every lab fell within the laboratory's suggested normal limits. That does not mean they are normal for her. First of all, 8–10% of people "normally" fall outside of normal limits, and secondly, define normal. She would not be in my office if everything were "normal."

Labs need to be interpreted from a bird's eye view. One must know the situation or concerns of the person we are doing labs on (that is why labs from health fairs are absolutely useless, especially when they are dropped off for a medical provider to interpret). One must see the forest to interpret the trees. Hormones, being messengers and very environmentally cued, need to have a "pattern." When one hormone is low normal, for example, another hormone being out of place (though still within normal limits) should cue a doctor into looking deeper or assuming fault or a problem. The deal should be sealed when, while looking at the labs, you know the patient's history and concerns. I cannot tell you the number of times a lab test says a hormone is normal, but the patient is telling me otherwise and, looking at all the hormones from that position above, all makes sense. That hormone is off for this person sitting in front of me.

This could be considered anecdotal medicine, but when the person sitting in front of you is at his or her rope's end, based on the findings and history, it should at least cue any caring doctor into further evaluation, at the least, or a trial of supplements, diet, or pre-scriptions at least. A detailed discussion of risks vs. benefits almost always ends with the patient being willing to accept any said risk, as the potential benefits could be life changing.

We had that very discussion and she, being a more conservatively bent person, decided on further or more advanced testing.

We started with a salivary diurnal cortisol test to check cortisol levels. (Author's comment: I wish I could get one of these competi-tors to do this test WHILE they are getting ready for a show or doing a Fat to Fit program). We also did a comprehensive gut analysis to look at the condition of her gut—a system that is destroyed by a Fat to Fit program.

The salivary cortisol levels showed low DHEA (a very import-ant hormone) and elevated cortisol levels that did not follow the God-directed curve of normalcy.

The gut test (or "poop" test as we call it in the office) showed high levels of inflammatory markers, low amounts of good bacteria in the gut, and poor absorption of fats and proteins.

We started our intervention with controlling the cortisol. I cut her workouts back to twice a week. This took some convincing, as exercise is good for you, right? I increased her calories and encour-aged her to take a night a week and really enjoy herself with food. I told her to get back to the dates with her husband, and to eat to her heart's content (I explain this later, don't worry). We started some supplements to lower cortisol and help with stress, such as Relora, L-Theanine, and Phosphorylated Serine (Seriphos®) before bed. I added Melatonin and asked her to stop all computers, texting, iPhones, IPads, and TV when the sun went down so her brain had a chance to rest and get ready for sleep.

We then worked on her gut by adding some digestive aids, and new probiotics, and I gave her several recipes for gut health, such as homemade yogurt, kimchi, and Kombucha. She already avoided processed foods, so that part was easy for her.

I warned her the process would be slow. Her quick results of the Fat to Fit program would not be experienced by her and, thanks to her good intellect and understanding, though disappointed, she understood and would be patient.

After about 4 months (sooner than most to be honest), she started to lose her belly fat. Her emotions leveled out. Her periods became lighter and her moods improved greatly. Over time, she returned to her original self. Not contest self, but HERSELF.

She was elated and thankful. She understood the process and the problem. She was back to who she, her husband, her kids, and her friends all loved. It took some time, but it was well worth it in her mind.

Since that time, she has become somewhat of an advocate against the Fat to Fit programs. She will walk up to people in the gym and offer a warning about what they are doing. She tells the trainers they are causing a problem. Most times it falls on deaf ears, but she won't stop. No one should have to suffer as she did, and her new mission is to help others avoid going through what she went through.

## The Yo-Yo

Jenny was a wonderful 32-year-old woman with success written all over her. A successful millennial if there ever was one, as she liked to brag. Successful in her career, successfully not married (her words), and a go-getter. She was 100% type A and, like me (we got along great!), had acronyms behind her name such as OCD and ADD, etc. These traits carried over into her constant desire (she would call it a need) to have the ultimate body. In her purse she carried an old photo of Rachel McLish—an early 1980s bodybuilder whom I remember quite well. Rachel had a muscular, but not grotesque body, with a lot of femininity. She was gorgeous, and she was who Jenny wanted to emulate. Jenny also had several photos on her phone of more recent figure models she was quick to review with me, not only to point out what she liked, but what she did not like or want.

The reason she came to see me was that, as all good type A or all-or-nothing people, she could diet with the best of them, but then crashed hard and regained weight like crazy. She was the type who, every time a new commercial for a weight loss or physique-modifying program came on the radio, cable TV, or social media—she bought it. Then she did it with more fervor than most could even hope for, but all of them eventually failed her. With some of them, she could not keep up the pace they required. Balancing work, social life, exercise and, on many occasions the strict eating plans, wore her down and her work life started to suffer. Not that she recognized it at first. She convinced herself she would not be weak and give in to her fatigue and foggy brain. Like other millennials, she felt she had something to prove and nothing was going to stop her. Two of the programs she tried, including one with a personal trainer doing CrossFit, caused injury that kept her out of the exercise game for some time. It did not matter to her. She was going to get a body like Rachel McLish. Period.

However, every time she felt she was getting close to that ideal physique, maybe 10 pounds away from it, she started to regain her weight, particularly in her belly and backside. Over the course of the previous year, she had approached that ideal look three different times, all within 10 pounds of perfect. The first time she came so close was with a home DVD set/program. She was rocking it hard— getting up at 0400 a.m. every day to get it done, working all day, and repeating it in the evening. She gained her weight back after the extreme fatigue took its toll. She had to quit the program and, being an all-or-nothing, she quit eating correctly as well. Her weight came back, and she felt it was due to her getting off the program. The second time, she lost it (or I should say gained it), she thought it was due to the injury she had suffered (mentioned above). She was no longer able to exercise and the weight came back with a vengeance.

The third time, that ideal look was just a few changes in the mirror away. Everything was going well, but the weight loss stopped and no matter what she did, the weight crept back on. She would exercise harder, eat less and less, but still gained weight. She felt it had to be hormonal. Something was off in her body, as she was doing everything perfectly, but that desired look was slipping farther and farther away. She was the classic yo-yo. That's when she made the appointment to see me.

As I mentioned above, we got along great. She was so much fun to talk to and get to know. She was a determined lady, and I was excited to get to know her better. We even compared the degree of our psychosis when it dealt with the OCD and ADD!

After hearing her story, I told her what she wanted to hear: her hormones were off. This would include her HPA Axis, her thyroid, her sex hormones—the works. This excited her, as she knew it! She immediately asked what we were going to do about it. I paused her and said I am not done yet—your gut is also jacked, the oxidative stress on your body is overwhelming, and you are a huge target for further weight gain and diseases in the not too distant future unless we make some changes. That part scared her. She was not the type to be scared either. She asked literally one-hundred questions and, being incredibly smart, she started to see the pattern of the Fat to Fit program I described.

She was a bit dazed at the end of her initial visit as she, like everyone who first sees the error of our Contemporary Diet and Exercise Recommendations, felt cheated. She admitted to being a bit down and depressed, but was willing to charge forward.

We decided to do hormonal testing that morning as she had not eaten and her menstrual cycle was off (it had been off for a few years since she had started her pursuit of the McLish body). We considered some oxidative stress labs, but I told her that, based on her history, they would all be positive (indicative of high oxidative stress), so we decided to save those, until we could see how she was progressing with the recovery program I would design for her.

I had her run over and see my dietitian for body composition and circumferential measurements, as well as to get her started on the *RecoverMe* eating plan (discussed in Chapter 10). I started her on the basic *RecoverMe* supplements following a Fat to Fit program (see Chapter 11), and waited for all her labs to come back to make it more individualized. I asked her to do nothing for exercise, but to go for a 30-min walk, outside in the sun, three to four times a week. She had a little issue with this, even after our long discussion, as she was convinced she would just gain more weight. I promised her that with everything we were in the process of doing, she would not lose any weight until we got her body fixed, but she would not gain anymore, either. She hesitantly agreed.

Her hormone labs came back a week later with all the typical Fat to Fit issues. Insulin was off, adiponectin was low, leptin was non-existent, testosterone was low, free T3 was low, DHEA was low, and cortisol was elevated.

Standard labs reveled elevated liver enzymes (meaning her liver was in trouble) and decreased kidney function—something I see in everyone who trains hard and uses a lot of protein powder.

With these findings, we decided to look a little deeper into her HPA axis, as she was the type who not only wanted to see more, but to understand it better. We ordered a diurnal salivary cortisol test. The results indicated some serious issues that needed addressed right away, but also encouraged us to do a little more.

We considered a gut test after reviewing the diurnal cortisol test, but decided just to treat her based on everything else.

She was started on very specific supplements for her condition, as the first step in her *RecoverMe* was to fix the HPA Axis. At the same time, I started some low dose thyroid medication, 7-KETO DHEA, and a cyclic progesterone at night to get her cycle back on track.

As I promised her when we discussed exercise, she would not have a McLish body right away, but she would stop gaining weight and start to feel better. I told her the most significant sign of **RecoverMe** was the way she felt—not body changes, not weight loss, but how her quality of life was affected. I also informed her that it would take at least three months to get her hormones all working again. Being a Type A, this was exactly three months too long but, once again, she trusted me and stuck to it.

At our follow-up which occurred about five months after our lab review visit, she stated that she had not felt this good in years as she had recently. She had not lost any weight yet but, as I had promised, she had not gained any either. Her periods had normalized, and she was sleeping well and felt really good. Her work life had improved incredibly, and she was due for a promotion. She was very excited and admitted the goals she had had for the McLish body were starting to fade. She still wanted to be in better shape, but the way she felt she would give that up to continue her current course.

The Yo-Yo dieting was done. She felt great on the **RecoverMe** eating plan and supplement schedule and had no intention of changing it. She stopped watching all the infomercials on weight loss programs. She stopped the Pinterest and Instagram feeds on motivation, weight loss, goals, and before and after pictures, as she realized these were feeding her psychosis. She only used social media to stay in contact with friends.

We discussed that as she changed—life situations, stressors, age, goals, etc.—we would need to change our intervention. Real life medicine is never static—it is dynamic. Doctors cannot prescribe a drug and plan on it for the rest of the person's life. That should be considered malpractice but, unfortunately, it is far too common.

We visited once again 6 months later and she was still doing great. She had started to drop weight, without even attempting to and was happy with her physique. She was not Rachel McLish, but she was Jenny! That was all that really mattered to her, as she was enjoying life to the fullest.

## Up 20+ Pounds in Menopause

Stacy was going through menopause. She stated that her first symptom to appear had been the gradual increase in her scale weight, even though she was an avid and aggressive exerciser and ate a strictly plant-based diet. Her periods started to become irregular, followed by the occasional hot flash and night sweat. Her OB/GYN told her that weight gain was normal and expected, but they could control the hot flashes and night sweats with a hormone called prempro (also known as a conjugated horse urine based estrogen and an artificial progestin called medroxyprogesterone acetate). She was going to have none of that. Taking artificial hormones was certainly out, and weight gain WAS NOT an option.

The solution: tough out the hot flashes and night sweats, increase her exercise, and lower her calories to lose the weight. She did just that, but to no avail. Exercising some days up to 3 to 4 hours, lifting weights, going to group classes, walking the dog, going on bike rides with friends—everything she could think of to increase her calorie usage, she did. Her already low-calorie diet went even more low calorie—under 1000 calories a day, still plant-based, and the weight kept creeping up.

With the increased exercise, she was starting to get achy all over and started relying on Advil before any exercise endeavor. Her sleep started to suffer as well, but she blamed this on night sweats, never relating it to the increased activity. It did strike her as odd, however, that she would go to bed so fatigued, but sleep terribly. She recalled that when first having night sweats, she could just fall back to sleep, but something was different now. Her mood and attitude toward life really started to suffer as well. No matter what she did, weight kept coming on. The more she tried to keep it off with her movement and eating, the more she gained.

She and her closest confidants all attributed it to hormones and "the change." That's how she made it to my clinic. She came in to discuss hormone replacement therapy, not realizing I would soon be discussing her eating and activity.

She was a very healthy "early 50ish" girl (that is all she would admit to until she realized I had her date of birth on my chart). She was lean and muscular, but quick to show me her belly and backside, where she claimed all the weight was going. We took her measurements and vitals and found that she was 20 pounds up from just six months earlier when this had all started. She was devastated. "How can anyone workout as hard as I do, and eat as little as I eat, and gain 20 pounds?" she asked. She then proceeded to answer her own question: "It's my hormones, right, Dr. Willey? Menopause does this to women, correct?"

I agreed with her, stating that was part of the problem, and likely the thing that had started the process. I then explained to her that we could also attribute some of the weight gain to her overzealous diet and exercise program. This one threw her for a loop, as she had always been able to lose any excessive weight with the same behaviors.

I then explained the concept of a Fat to Fit program and what it does to the body—hormones included. I also helped her understand that when one undertakes a Fat to Fit program, with hormones already in distress (in her case menopause), things really go south quickly—hence the 20 pounds in such a short time. The more I explained the problem, the effects on the gut, the oxidative stress, and the hormonal disarray, the more sense it started to make to her.

Our intervention started with balancing her hormones. We obtained the appropriate labs and studies, and replaced all her sex hormones in the appropriate amounts and delivery methods. I also started her on some supplements and continued her on her plant-based eating plan, but made sure her protein was adequate and she was eating enough for her body as per **RecoverMe**.

It took some convincing to have her cut back on her exercise, and honestly—I don't think she did the first few months of our intervention. I teased her about it at our 3-month follow-up, but she never admitted to me whether or not she was still doing it. No matter—she was doing much better. We had taken care of her hot flashes and night sweats. Her moods improved, sex life was good, and she was feeling better. The weight was slow to come off and she was still not sleeping that well, even though she was having no more night sweats or hot flashes. This was my opportunity to encourage her to cut back a little on her exercise so her body would recover and repair itself—that is, lower the stress hormone, sleep better, and let the fat go.

At our six-month follow-up, she was down ten pounds from our initial visit and was sleeping better. She had finally backed off on her exercise, and found it left a lot more time for other things like family and friends. She was very excited. Her only concern was some vaginal dryness during sex, so we made some hormone adjustments after obtaining some labs.

A year later, she was in cruise mode. She was at her ideal weight, feeling good, and without complaints. Her diet was steady and more than she had ever eaten in the past. She only went to the gym or participated in group classes three times a week now—a huge change from when we met. On the days when she did not go to the gym, she went on walks and/or bike rides with her family and friends, or just worked in her yard, weather permitting. She continued a few of the supplements I originally suggested, as she stated she could tell they were doing their job because, when she ran out of them, she knew it.

I informed her that it was/is a really good idea to continue regular follow-ups and lab checks with me. As we get wiser (older), our bodies change, and I help adjust the hormones, supplements, diet, and exercise to adapt to those changes. Being proactive in health always triumphs over being reactive—and she could not have agreed more.

## The Ex-College Athlete (as told by her)

www.ashleyrayfit.com

"College athlete" is often times a misunderstood lifestyle, full of stereotypes and preconceived notions. What follows is my personal story entailing the stresses of the day-to-day life of a college student, in combination with being a college athlete, and what it did to me mentally and physically.

Growing up in a very competitive household and watching my older siblings compete in various sports encouraged me to be just like them. Being the youngest in my family, and having my father as a coach, I wanted nothing more than to be successful and earn a college softball scholarship. Having my father as a coach was the best thing I could ever have asked for. He helped me train nonstop for college, which made me think I was mentally and physically prepared for anything.

My freshman year of college was much like that of any other freshman, I suppose. I was scared, excited, and ready to start a new chapter in my life. Even though I felt prepared for college, I could never have guessed the stress incurred by a collegiate athlete. It was more responsibility than I even knew existed. Immediately, we were thrown into non-stop meetings, early morning workouts, strenuous practices, and hours of study hall in order to keep our grades up. Not to mention, I was lucky if I got 5 hours of sleep a night.

For the first two years of college, we had a two-week rotation of practice hours. For two weeks, we would have weights from 4:00 a.m. to 6:00 a.m., heating and stretching from 1:00 p.m. to 2:00 p.m., practice from 2:30 p.m. to 5:30 p.m., time spent with the trainers post-practice (more heating, icing, stretching, and massaging) 5:30

p.m. to 6:30 p.m. Along with that, a typical weekday consisted of 45 minutes to 1 hour to eat dinner and then head to our team-required study hall from 7:30 p.m. to 9:00 p.m.

After two weeks, we would switch to 11:00 p.m. to 2:00 a.m. practice hours and weights and conditioning from 3:00 p.m. to 5:00 p.m. To deal with my stress, I often found myself in the gym off campus. I have always loved to lift weights and eat healthy. The gym and eating right was my "happy" place. However, overexercising and undereating can cause Athlete's Triad Syndrome, which I had battled with once in high school. It made a triumphant return during my freshman year of college. I experienced several injuries and illnesses, such as strained back, pulled muscles, walking pneumonia, tonsillitis, mononucleosis, and was constantly battling colds, sore throats and exhaustion.

After completing two years at my first college, I knew it wasn't the place for me. With my dad's help that following summer (after having my tonsils removed), I found my passion again for softball and tried out for the US International Softball Team.

I played for a short period of time in the Dominican Republic. Although I had a blast and experienced the best thing any athlete can ever dream of, I lost around 10 pounds and only weighed 110 pounds when I returned to the States. A week after returning, I walked onto the Idaho State University campus and softball team, where I finished my last 2 years of college.

The experience here, however, was very similar to that of my first two years of college. Constant traveling, training, lifting, and long practices. Being a college athlete is, without a doubt, a full-time job that is emotionally and physically draining. However, as any athlete would most likely explain, there is a love and passion for sports and the constant roller coaster and exhaustion are a part of the "game." You may think I'm odd, but being the competitive person I am, I loved being pushed to my limits most of the time.

While playing D1 collegiate softball, I still managed to find myself in the gym outside of team practices and weights/conditioning. I have always been a very picky eater and did not eat the calories my body needed for the amount of training I was doing. Because of this, I constantly battled having regular monthly cycles, which impacted my energy, strength, and mood. I was put on medication to prevent osteoporosis and tried several different types of birth control to help regulate my body. With the excessive training, I was constantly battling muscle soreness, fatigue, and emotional instability.

Going into our first tournament of my senior season, I dove for a fly ball, landing awkwardly, breaking both my radius and ulna, and tearing my patellar tendon. These led to arm and knee surgery, ending my softball career. I still continued on to graduate with my bachelors.

That following summer was emotionally wearing due to a few family losses. I spent most my time recovering from my surgery and injuries, and was later diagnosed with West Nile Virus. This took several months to bounce back from. That fall I started graduate school and began my internship with the amazing Dr. Willey.

During this time, I was in a very toxic relationship, and managed to hide it very well from those around me. In my two years of graduate school I was very adamant about wanting to compete in bodybuilding. Again, I used the gym as my outlet for the stress brought on by this toxic relationship and school. To help control the weight and body fat I had gained, Dr. Willey had me try various diets, workouts, and hormone treatments. It seemed as if, no mat-ter what I did, I was gaining body fat while also being emotionally exhausted and constantly being put down in the relationship I was in. I went months without sugar, re-feed (cheat) meals, or any type of relaxation whatsoever. I then came to a breaking point. Mentally and physically, I was in a very rough place. It helped me completely understand what many athletes go through after college, with regard to fighting weight gain.

Toward the end of graduate school, I went through several months of different court hearings due to the relationship I was in. I also endured another surgery, but managed to stay very dedicated to my diet and wanted to get back on track to a healthier life in every way. I soon realized I was being stubborn and was not truly listening to Dr. Willey's advice. I always knew he was right, my mind just couldn't overcome that the gym was my release!

I began to consume more calories, staying very low carbohydrate and particularly higher in fats and proteins. I spent the next two and a half years patiently waiting for results. I knew through his experience, words of wisdom, and hormone treatments I would eventually level out again. After about two years of following his diet regimen and exercise advice, I brought in more "cheat" meals. I really started to enjoy food again and life in general. My attitude started to change for the better. I eventually tapered off the hormone treatment and began noticing changes in my body fat and weight measurements.

It has now been three years since I graduated school and a year and half free of hormone therapy. I am currently back down to the weight and body fat I was at in college, but feel drastically different and significantly healthier. I am still very passionate about the gym and living a healthy lifestyle. I've learned that recovering from excessive overtraining and undereating takes a lot of time, dedication, and consistency.

The amount of mental, physical, and emotional stress affected me to a great extent. Although I made collegiate sports seem as if they were nothing but misery, certain parts also brought me the best experience I could ever ask for. I love being an athlete. If I could give any words of advice to young athletes, they would be to train wisely, feed your body, and always remember it is better to be under-trained than overtrained. Rest is a critical part of being an athlete, as well as eating the amount of calories your body needs.

For those who are battling the "postcollege sport weight gain," I encourage you to be very patient in your time of recovery. Try your best to keep a positive attitude, as hard as it may be, and allow your body and mind the time they need to recuperate. It's not going to happen overnight, or maybe even over the course of the first year, but it will happen. I can't stress enough that it takes time, effort and the right amount of relaxation. Without this time, effort and recovery, even the most comprehensive workouts, supplements, and dieting will not improve an overtrained athlete's overall wellness.

**Author's Observations:**

I asked Ashley to provide her comments for a few reasons. The first being, Ashely was a classic ex-athlete like those I see all the time. Dedicated, sure of herself, confident, but due to the Fat to Fit nature of her training, she was set up for eventual failure. The second reason is she worked with me daily for years. It is so hard to understand the problems with the Fat to Fit mentality, that even being side-by-side most days of the week, it took a ton of convincing, almost three years, for her to finally listen and let me help her fix the underlying Fat to Fit issue. She was seeing us treat the issues in others, but it was hard for her to see it in herself. Before I convinced her to follow the healing regimen I designed, she witnessed herself getting fatter—so being in the field and knowing what to do, she exercised harder and ate less—doing nothing but making the problems worse. She understood the fallacies of modern dieting and the relationship of stress and hormonal issues caused by said dieting, but it still took her almost three years to recover and fix herself. How much harder may it be for everyone out there reading this to believe me and the issues with a Fat to fit program, when my co-worker and friend took so long to see it? My hope is it does not take you as long as it did my good friend Ashley.

Our interventions with Ashley are like those I describe later in the ***RecoverMe*** section of this book. The first thing we did is decrease cortisol via stress control. One of the biggest components of stress control? Decrease the amount and intensity of exercise and start feeding her body what it needed to thrive, not just survive. We worked on sleep and mindful meditation, and utilized supplements to help decrease the hormonal disarray. We used some hormone replacement therapy to act as a bridge for her obvious deficiency. The deficiency, by the way, was in her story and appearance, as the lab's values were not that far off.

Focusing on lowering the cortisol, optimizing the other hormones negatively affected by the high-stress state, made all the difference in the world for Ashley. It cannot be emphasized enough, that modern thinking of "more is better" when it comes to exercise and "less is better" when it comes to food, is the major contributor to all the fitness failures out there. Ashley provides us with yet one more example of this inborn error within a Fat to Fit program.

## For the Long Haul

Debbie was a 28-year-old endurance athlete. She loved doing the big races—Spartan races and marathons. She was built for it. Tall and lean with a stride that was the envy of her competitors. She had always been a runner, running cross-country in high school and college, but took a little time off (about 8 months) to get married and relocate due to her husband's new job. When she got settled, she was right back out pounding the streets. She had her own training style, but loved to try new ones. She was constantly on the Internet endurance blogs and web sites trying all sorts of different training regimens. Her goal was to run at least 8 miles a day, most days a week. Most of the time she got a lot more mileage in, but she never went below 8 miles a day. She had done a couple of marathons in the preceding months before meeting with me and was in the process of training for an Iron Woman event.

She was referred to me by a fellow runner who had seen me a few years earlier for the same issue she was experiencing of recent. She and her husband had been trying to conceive for the last year with no luck. She had all the conventional testing via her OB/GYN and had a referral in hand for a fertility clinic, but she wanted to try a less costly and more natural approach. While I am not a fertility specialist, I help a lot of families get kids. My staff likes to joke about the fact we tend to get girls pregnant all the time. Getting people healthy is our secret, and understanding the hormones involved helps. A little!

Upon meeting and getting a detailed history, she shared a few more issues that I found very telling. Her periods had stopped. She could not shake a darn cold she had been dealing with for months. She felt foods of all kinds were irritating her belly, so she could not figure out what to eat. She could not get out of a mental funk she described as being down. A little depressed and anxious with no reason to be sad or worried. Her marriage was great, finances were good, she felt her training for her Iron Woman was going well (other than being more fatigued this time then previously), and she wanted a baby. With these things, my history-taking revealed that she felt her recovery time was lengthening. It was taking longer to heal, especially her legs, than it had before. She was experiencing a lot more cramps, having a hard time stretching, and had a couple of hamstring issues she had never had to deal with in all her running career. She described her legs as feeling heavy. These concerns were not enough to stop her, just irritating.

Her physical exam was, by most standards, normal. But I found a few things that raised my eyebrows. She was extremely lean, but incredibly soft. She had no muscle tone. Her reflexes where quicker than expected. Her ankles and feet had a tiny bit of edema. I did her body comp and the numbers were significantly higher than would be expected by looking at her. Here thyroid was a little large but otherwise normal, and she had a little bit of lower belly fat that one would not expect for the amount of exercise she did. Nothing major, but all adding up.

We had a great discussion as to what was going on, but we obtained some early morning labs to confirm it. Since we could not mark her time of the month via her period, we guessed it based on changes in vaginal discharge.

Her labs came back with the following concerns:

1. She was mildly anemic (low blood counts) likely due to #2
2. Iron stores were very low
3. Androgens (testosterone and DHEA) were low
4. Cholesterol panel was off
5. Her thyroid function was less than optimal
6. Estrogen, progesterone, and the brain hormones FSH and LH were all low (if we were correct on the time of month, it should not have been this way)
7. RBC Mg+ levels were very low
8. She had a lot of eosinophils in her complete blood count (CBC)
9. Kidney function was less than optimal as her GFR was elevated

GFR stands for Glomerular Filtration Rate. It is a marker of kidney function. When GFR is high, it can indicate low muscle mass, poor nutrition, chronic illness, etc. Debbie was the classic Fat to Fit person with the clinical presentation and all the labs to match. Her under-recovery (not overtraining—see Chapter 9) from all her activity, poor/undereating and all the stress it had created in her body set her up for her status. Not only was she feeling bad and not able to compete as she wanted to, she was in no way, shape, or form going to get pregnant in this current state.

As we reviewed the labs and all the suggested interventions, the one that was most difficult for her to grasp was cutting back on her exercise. Like others before her, that is one that challenges too many classic paradigms as modern and historical thinking has been "more is better."

After convincing her to cut back on exercise, I had her visit with my dietitian to help her increase her protein and caloric intake, optimize gut function, and avoid possible food allergies/triggers with her complaints of not being able to eat anything of recent. I started her on a few supplements to increase iron, vitamins, and mineral levels, in particular, magnesium. We agreed to watch her thyroid closely as we considered making some adjustments.

I started her on cyclic progesterone and testosterone consisting of low dose testosterone replacement daily along with daily progesterone with the dosing changes mid-month to mimic/restart her menstrual cycles. I separated the compounded hormones, as my experience had been when young ladies like her initiate our intervention, they tend to get pregnant rather quickly. I informed her to stop the testosterone if she did get pregnant and talk to her OB doctor about the progesterone when she met with her.

At our three-month follow up, Debbie could not be happier. She felt great again, was running regularly, but not excessively, had put on some good muscle mass—she was up 10 pounds, but stated she and her husband loved the way she looked. She looked "lean and mean" not soft and flat anymore. She stated her periods started to return the first month of intervention, and the week before our meeting, she had a full regular cycle. This was very exciting to her as she knew she could get pregnant now. We check a few labs and they showed her RBC Mg+ levels had normalized as had her iron stores and her anemia and kidney issue had normalized. I had her continue all her current interventions with plans for a six month follow up.

About 10 weeks later, I got an email from her stating she would not be following up with me at our six-month appointment. She was pregnant and could not be more thankful and excited. She had scheduled an appointment with her OB as we discussed!

Debbie is now a full time stay-at-home mom with not just one child, but three! I still see her on a regular basis as she considers me her accountability doctor to keep her exercise in control. She completely resolved and fixed her Fat to Fit issues and lifestyle. I would bet money on the fact she will never return to it.

The next few paragraphs are written by my medical assistant, Lisa, from her point of view of our common and very wonderful patients.

## My Classic Patient (as told by my medical assistant)

Brick by Brick

Ten years ago, I walked into a medical office in Pocatello and I met Dr. Willey. I was absolutely terrified of him! This medical office was having a very busy day and I shook hands with this strange doctor and he asked me about me, about my skills, and then disappeared for the rest of the day seeing patients. I was a brand new Medical Assistant, entering my first job, I wasn't too confident of my skills and then I was asked to jump into the deep end of the pool and swim by a doctor. It scared me.

Today, I am still with this office; however, my fear of Dr. Willey has disappeared. I am sure I just annoy him now. The good doctor is very patient with me, though, and is even so good as to teach me what is in that head of his. One thing I asked him to teach me more about was hormone therapy and I truly appreciate the opportunity to learn this cool facet of human physiology.

As we work together, we meet several types of folks who come to Dr. Willey with very similar complaints. One of the most common types of patients we see are men and women with hormone concerns and weight issues. They fit a typical constitution: usually they are about 45 or so, with complaints of fatigue, trouble losing weight and lack of sex drive. They feel frustrated as they tell about why they are being seen: because nothing that used to work for their complaints works any more. They've tried eating less and exercising more and are trying to eat healthier, but the tiredness, weight gain, and hormone issues persist. They are totally stumped about the sex drive; they just want it fixed, as they all claim they have great relationships with their loved ones.

I check them in and take their histories and then the good doctor comes in and he chats with them. He listens patiently, averages around 45 to 60 minutes with each of them and shares his knowledge with them, just as he has with me. Then he steps out and asks me to go in and "swipe their blood." The order will be basic hormone labs such as a total testosterone, estradiol, a basic thyroid workup, maybe some brain hormones, and some basic chemistries. I let the patient know the labs will be back quickly and, as soon as Dr. Willey has reviewed them, I will call them to review the results.

In a day or two, the labs are back and I am on the phone, chatting with them about lab results. Occasionally, they feel frustrated because the labs look good. Dr. Willey didn't find any obvious abnormalities in the labs and the patient was hoping they would shed a little light on why he/she doesn't feel like his or her self. I ask the patient to please come back and follow up with Dr. Willey for the next steps. Upon follow up, Dr. Willey shows them that although the lab values are "within normal limits" they still validate their concerns. He focuses on personalized recovery programs including more detailed diagnostic procedures and testing, dietary recommendations, and proper supplements, and cleans up their medication lists. Dr. Willey knows which medications are weight positive and weight negative and he understands how important diet is to health. The face-to-face chats are vital to addressing tender things like sexual health. The human body is an amazing thing, and under proper care, it thrives.

It's interesting to see these patients. I enjoy the science of the hormone cascade and drawing blood and learning about the physiology of the human body. I enjoy learning at the foot of a doctor who lets me annoy him and learn from him at the same time. I love watching patients succeed who are their own advocates and are willing to listen to the good doctor and learn from him. The ones who succeed are the ones who can see the larger picture and are patient with their bodies being fixed. The ones who realize Dr. Willey is trying to teach them a basic lifestyle change. It is as Hadrian, a Roman Emperor, told his soldiers, "Brick by brick, my citizens, brick by brick."

## CHAPTER SUMMARY

Do you fit into one of these six case examples? Are there any aspects of these case examples that are descriptive of you or your situation? Chances are rather high, I would guess, if you are reading this book.

I could have added many more examples of people who have suffered from the modern diet and exercise recommendations. There are so many ways it shows up in doctors' offices around the world but are unfortunately missed as we are so ingrained into thinking that **ALL** low calorie eating and intense exercise is good for us. We must change the modern thinking in our modern environment.

The next few chapters will review **WHY** our current diet and exercise recommendations are so flawed for today's world.

# PART II
## Summary of Modern Diet and Exercise Programs and Their Problems

Before I go into a little more detail of the flaws of most of the diet and exercise programs out there being suggested and utilized, I want to give you a quick summary of what these programs do to you, then follow it with a review of what I consider to be the three primary problems with them.

If I were to summarize my goal for you in understanding all the popular and employed diet and exercise programs, it would be this: all of the diets, exercise plans, supplements, and drugs, have a common theme of high cortisol levels/stress levels. This plays a major role in and has effects on all the other hormones and metabolic activity in your body.

Current and popular diet and exercise programs increase something we call Allostatic Load or, simply put, repetitive damage or destruction of the mind and body. It is caused by continuing harmful activity (stresses) that challenges the body and mind's normal adaptation capability. As the body attempts to adapt to the Allostatic Load of a modern diet and exercise program, it starts to fail and the physiologic consequences of this adapting to repeated or chronic stress can fast-track disease processes and, in general, make you really feel terrible.

This Allostatic Load is remembered by the body very well—in other words: next time it sees it, it protects against it and mechanisms are in place that appear to prevent you from doing it again. Ever wonder why the low to no carb diet worked the first time but not again?

The exercise, the eating plans, the supplements and drugs all cause excessive stress/cortisol, which has many downstream issues including:

- Decreased immune system response to disease
- Increased immune response to self (autoimmune disease)
- Lowering of the sex hormones and growth hormone
- Increased fat in the belly (abdominal/visceral adiposity)
- Increased blood pressure
- Cognitive decline ("fuzzy brain")
- Muscle wasting
- Bone wasting
- Sugar cravings
- Salt cravings
- Depression/anxiety
- Insomnia
- Mood issues (quick to anger)
- Fatigue
- Dizziness
- Insulin resistance
- Increased inflammation
- Skin changes including acne

- And many more

This list describes the exact opposite of what the all the current diet and exercise programs are supposed to do! As you work for that new body, doing one of these programs, you're not only supposed to look good, but feel good, sleep better, have a better sex life, get a raise at work, never fight with your spouse again, drive a new car, and several other claims made by exercise and/or diet programs out there.

The exercise and diet program, over time and/or as a result, does just the opposite of what it was supposed to do. In the short term, a few may succeed—bodybuilders, fitness or physique artists, etc.—but in reality, everyone eventually pays the Piper, unless it is done correctly and in the right time frame for your body to adapt to the work/stress load.

Once you understand the problems associated with the current and popular thinking, I will cover how to do two things:

1. Recover from it
2. Prevent it from happening again

The next few pages will give you more detail on the three main tenets or problems of a modern exercise and diet program:

1. Problem 1—The Exercise
2. Problem 2—The Diet
3. Problem 3—The Supplements and the Drugs

# CHAPTER 4
## Problem 1–Too Much Exercise

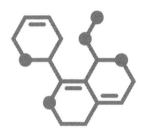

Reviewing the obvious, any sort of fitness-related goal, such as bodybuilding or any physique-related activity requires exercise. Even if you're just trying to get in shape or be healthy, it requires exercise. Not your walk in the park exercise, but intense, grilling, detailed and, more often than not, painful exercise. Every motivational poster, saying, and fitness/health related Pinterest out there tells you that you are not achieving your goal because you are not working hard enough. Every person who has made it to the fitness hall of fame, or just looks good in the gym or naked, is not shy in telling you how hard they worked to obtain and maintain that desired physique. You have been inundated with the idea that you can get that body you want **IF** you train hard enough. You are also told that if you do not get that body you are after, it is your fault! You, my dear friend, did not train hard enough!

So, what do you do? You train really hard. And when you see it not working, you train harder. You change your schedule so you can get an extra hour in the gym. You put aside your job, your friendships, and even your family, as nothing is going to stop you from looking like that girl/guy in the magazine. Your entire life starts revolving around working out. Sound familiar? Almost all the "body-obtaining" programs out there encourage this. Obvious or not, they are inspiring it. To the point of idolatry, you exercise your life away.

Some may be asking, "What's wrong with that? I thought and have always been told exercise is good for you?" Well…yes, it is. But moderation is better. Let me explain. Part of the reason you basically remain fat even when you are fit is that you dive right into this program you read about or saw on Dr. Oz full bore, without taking into consideration long-term consequences. In other words, what these programs profess is, at a basic physiological level, bad for you.

When you go from fat to fit, it involves a tremendous amount of exercise and effort. This exercise and effort are very stressful on your body. Cortisol, the stress hormone, skyrockets with this sort of training and, over time, starts wreaking havoc on your entire system. Exercise-related increases in cortisol response can be compared to the death of a loved one. How, you may ask? Think of it this way: from the neck down, cortisol is cortisol. Your body can't tell the difference nor does it know why it is elevated. From the neck up, your brain makes a distinction between good and bad. The death of a loved one = bad. Exercise = good. To your body = both are the same. Both cause severe stress and all the mental, physiologic, and emotional damage. This is just part of the reason you are Fat Also Fit. To top it off, your restrictive diet is making matters worse—I will cover that in the next section. Just know it is compounded by this lifestyle.

I think it important that I cover the body's stress response here so you can understand some of the interventions I cover later in the *RecoverMe* section. I will readdress this in Chapter 8 under **HPA Axis Adversity.**

Being in a high-stress situation, like the two plus hours you spend in the gym doing a modern exercise program, results in the release of increased levels of cortisol from the adrenal cortex. This release of cortisol is dictated by the paraventricular nucleus of the hypothalamus in the brain, where corticotropin-releasing hormone (CRH) is released in response to the stress. CRH then tells the pituitary gland to release adrenocorticotrophic hormone (ACTH) which, in turn, causes the adrenal cortex to release cortisol.

CRH and ACTH are released in short bursts, and each causes a sustained release of cortisol from the adrenal cortex. Cortisol's primary role is releasing glucose into the bloodstream to initiate the "flight or fight" response. It also suppresses and modifies the immune system, reproductive system, and digestive system.

During normal, non-stress situations, a certain level of cortisol is maintained in the bloodstream. There is a circadian rhythm of ACTH and cortisol release, with the highest levels occurring in the morning (roughly 0800 hours) and the lowest levels sometime early evening/evening (person dependent). The circadian pattern of cortisol release is controlled by the suprachiasmatic nucleus (SCN) of the hypothalamus. Signals from the SCN cause the paraventricular nucleus (PVN) of the hypothalamus to release pulses of CRH roughly once per hour, resulting in HPA axis activation and cortisol release. There are also direct links between the SCN and the adrenal gland itself, through sympathetic nerve fibers. Other hormones released by the hypothalamus also follow a circadian rhythm. Growth hormone release peaks during sleep, and melatonin is released at night.

Stress, such as intense exercise, causes an increased overall cortisol output. During chronic stress, changes occur in the neurons in the PVN and other areas in the brain, resulting in increased sustained activation of the HPA axis. Stress lasting longer than a few weeks can result in negative feedback to the HPA axis, causing a number of further issues (time is actually very person dependent—one person can get in a chronic stress mode in a matter of days and others may take weeks). Chronic stress results in high or low cortisol output, depending on several variables including how long you have been doing the up-to-date diet and exercise program, the degree of your involvement, and your body's response to the situation.

Another system in the body adversely affected by the extremes o f exercise is the autonomic nervous system. It consists of two branches: the sympathetic system and the parasympathetic system. The sympathetic nervous system is triggered during any type of physical or mental stress. It causes your heart rate and blood pressure to increase. It reduces heart rate variability (HRV) to keep the heart steady (read how to test HRV as a measure of your body's stress in Chapter 8), stops digestion, and centralizes blood flow. The parasympathetic nervous system has the opposite effect: it reduces heart rate and blood pressure, increases heart rate variability, and facilitates/allows digestion. The sympathetic system and the parasympathetic system are working in balance: when sympathetic activation is high, parasympathetic nervous activation is reduced, and when the parasympathetic system is active, the sympathetic system is decreased. Under normal conditions, the sympathetic nervous system is activated during stress and the parasympathetic system is more active during the recovery phase after the stress.

While doing a currently recommended program, the sympathetic system tends to stay in high gear, while parasympathetic activity is reduced. Interestingly, studies have indicated that lack of parasympathetic activity correlates with feelings of fatigue.

Defining fatigue is also difficult for people to understand. Research has shown that fatigue is, in fact, an emotion created in the brain. This emotions appears to sense that further exposure to the stress that created it will cause additional damage to the body and mind. It appears to be protective. Several other body factors related to extremes of exercise, like those in a modern exercise program, are also involved in fatigue: muscle soreness, core body temperature and rate of heat accumulation, glycogen (energy) levels in the muscles, oxygen levels in the brain, thirst, sleep deprivation, etc. Psychological factors such as motivation, baseline emotional state, and knowledge of the endpoint also add to the well-defined fatigue.

What this means is that the brain perceives the problem with your exercise program early on. The combination of physical, mental, and emotional factors generates this "emotion" we call fatigue, in an attempt to slow you down and recover. Unfortunately, at the heart of all popular programs is the underlying belief that fatigue, soreness, and being worn-out are good things and are supposed to happen! The exercise portion of these programs also tells you (as do all the silly motivational posters/sayings out there) that if you do not ignore this emotion, you are a wimp and not worthy of a new body.

The intense, stress-producing exercise plus the diet and supplements (or drugs) of these programs all compound. In some individuals, the autonomic dysfunction and severe fatigue, occurs at a much lower than expected level of intensity. This means you do not have to run a marathon to obtain this problem. It may happen with a 5k or even just training for a 5k. That causes confusion and difficulty for a doctor trying to figure out why these healthy-looking people feel so bad (See Part III, Chapter 8 on the Medical Evaluation).

The majority of people under this scenario, rebound after getting close to or obtaining their goal. Your body literally says, "Hell no! I am done and I am **NOT** doing that again." You lose 25 pounds to hit your goal, but your vigorous cortisol raising exercise is part of the reason you gain those 25 pounds back and add 10 more. High cortisol levels also cause water retention via another hormone called aldosterone—one of the reasons your weight can go up and down so quickly in this scenario. It is your body's protective mechanism. You have literally doomed yourself to failure in the long run. There are, of course, exceptions. We all know and see them. Guys and gals who train hard all the time and look good. There are three possible scenarios in this case: 1. They are on drugs that combat or at very least balance the cortisol chaos and metabolic changes that occur with overly intense exercise; 2. they are genetically gifted to handle it; 3. they have adapted the lifestyle that allows control of the stress hormones and their recovery is optimal. We, of course, want number three, and that is what we will be covering in detail later. If it is just the drugs, have no fear; they will get theirs later. You cannot do drugs forever without consequences, and genetics can be overridden by a rotten lifestyle, eventually.

The physiologic chemistry of a person doing or having done a popular diet and exercise program is not unlike that of the sick population. Some cases I have seen are not unlike that of a person in the hospital! They have several metabolic changes including blood sugar issues, endocrine and hormonal issues, increased levels of lactic acid in their systems, water and electrolyte imbalances, nutrient depletion that sets one up for disease states, and body composition changes that are not in the direction they want! People who only use the scale never see it (so they are happy and thinking they are doing well with their program, not realizing it's a metabolic warning signal), but those who do body composition will see increasing fat and loss of lean mass—the exact opposite of what they are after.

Others may have excessive fat loss with this type of training. Is it possible to have excessive fat loss? I thought that was what we were after, Doc? Well, yes, it is possible. You can lose your fat too quickly—when you consider the big picture. I have seen it many times and get into actual arguments with clients when I want them to slow down. It will backfire on you, trust me. Look at "the Biggest Loser" contestants. How many of them have maintained their weight/fat loss? Part of their problem with their fat to fit, televised program is this very issue.

Intense exercise also causes something called endotoxemia. Endotoxemia basically means toxins in the blood. The term was coined originally in/for animals, based on a certain type of bacteria being present and releasing a toxin. Now we know different forms of endotoxemia can occur when the gut breaks down.

Lipopolysaccharide or LPS is one way to measure if endotoxemia is present/occurring (listed under oxidative stress markers below).

The negative hormonal changes that occur with excessive training/exercise programs are quite impressive. It is far beyond the scope of this book to cover them all, but let me just mention a few of them in this next section.

## The Negative Effect of an Excessive Exercise Program on Your Hormones

We have discussed the elevation of cortisol with the excessive exercise programs. High cortisol levels increase something called reverse T3 (rT3). T3 or triiodothyronine is the active thyroid hormone. Your brain produces thyroid-stimulating hormone (TSH) to tell your thyroid (a little butterfly-shaped gland in your neck) to produce the thyroid hormones T4 and T3 (simplified). T4 could be considered the inactive thyroid hormone, as the body removes an iodine from it to make the active thyroid hormone T3. T3 then does all the wonderful things you have heard about, including energy and heat regulation, brain function, and a list of beneficial and important things longer than this page. Reverse T3 literally stops T3 from doing its work. In other words, your modern, hard-core exercise program causes thyroid dysfunction. Your thyroid function looks normal on paper (so says your doctor), but you feel awful, are losing hair, getting fatter, and know your thyroid is off. When you can finally no longer do your excessive exercising, this really puts you in a bad place. That was too soft—this fact absolutely messes you up in the end!

Testosterone is also unfavorably affected. Testosterone is vital in both men and women for building muscle, burning fat, mood, energy, sense of well-being, and sexual drive and function. One overdone, overly excessive exercise session lowers your testosterone for up to 4 days. Your modern diet and exercise program has you training daily. Do the math—you're in trouble. It's not just compounded, it's exponential! So, the popular suggested training lowers your testosterone and increases cortisol, as I described above. This adversely affects something called your testosterone/cortisol ratio. This is a very important ratio and with crazy modern exercise programs, the ratio of the two goes in the wrong direction. The higher the ratio (high testosterone, low cortisol) the better the training gains and success. The lower the ratio (low testosterone, high cortisol), training gains literally cease. Your workouts aren't doing squat (even if you're squatting!). But wait! There is more: High cortisol lowers free testosterone, in part by increasing sex hormone binding globulin (SHBG) so even the testosterone you have is not working! Dang—that is not good. More importantly, there will be consequences down the road for this ratio being off.

Due to the excessive exercise effects on the body, a large number of people use drugs to help combat them. Therefore, the most popular drugs in the physique perfecting world are anabolic steroids, testosterone, and the thyroid hormone T3 (drug example: Cytomel). The current dogma training regimen ruins your testosterone/cortisol ratio. People are not about to train lighter or less to lower cortisol and increase testosterone, because Pinterest said they would be an enormous loser if they did. So what do people do? They take testosterone or other anabolic steroids to change the ratio with no mind to long-term consequences. They also use T3, especially if they are getting ready for an event, such as a physique show, as higher levels help combat the effects of elevated rT3. Once again, not without consequences.

Extreme exercise also does terrible things to one's mind and emotions. It changes your brain. High cortisol causes degeneration of the hippocampus—the area for memory; the hypothalamus—the part of your brain responsible for chronic fatigue syndrome, fibromyalgia, depression, and post-traumatic stress disorder; the prefrontal cortex—the area for executive decision making; and finally the amygdala—the part of your brain responsible for emotional stability.

Did any of those descriptive words raise your eyebrows? Anyone reading this feel any of these? Or gone to your doctor with the complaints of poor memory, extreme fatigue, body aches, depression, and emotional liability, such as yelling at the kids or spouse for no reason? And don't forget no sex drive and poor function. Don't worry—your doctor will give you an antidepressant. Yeah, that will work!

Some of these changes are permanent—scary eh? Pathological changes can be seen on a functional MRI (fMRI) when this situation is occurring. I keep referring to long-term consequences. Here is a big one. Your trend-setting training program shrank and changed your brain! Wow! "Wow" and "Oh crud" at the same time.

Your body does give you a warning sign, however. Besides the above-mentioned concerns, you become physically exhausted, but referring to what I said before—it never once crosses your mind that you are doing it to yourself with the exercise program. Oh no… it can't be that (how many times I have heard this in clinical practice). People swear it is their busy schedule, or a relationship issue, or they are fatigued from playing taxi for their four kids, all in different sports, etc. It is never the exercise, because remember—that's good for you! Unfortunately, if I may throw a clinical commentary out there: the busy schedule, the relationship issues, etc. are part of the picture, but the extreme exercise is compounding it. I have seen relationships heal and resolve when the body goals were dropped. Schedules relax when you don't have to spend 3 hours in the gym each day. In other words, there is a cure for this – it's just not an easy one, especially for those of us mental on and about our bodies.

That brings us to the next problem with Fat To Fit programs: the diet. This is a huge problem; arguably bigger than the exercise phenomenon I have described above. It is certainly additive to the exercise, as the eating is of absolute importance for recovery from the exercise, seconded only by sleep.

# CHAPTER 5

## Problem 2–Too Little Eating (or) Get the Body I Want NOW Eating

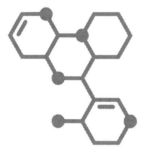

"Every diet works for somebody, but no diet works for everybody." This is likely very true, but when one starts a voguish exercise and/or diet program and it is their first attempt at getting leaner, with less body fat and more muscle, it tends to work for everyone. Hence, its popularity. The developers and spokespersons for the diet bank on this fact. When approached as to why it did not work a second or third time, the answer mimics the Pinterest Motivation page: "It's your fault, you cheated on the diet, you're a failure. It is not the pro-gram's fault!"

The second try, after the fat has shown itself again fails a large majority of people who had success the first time. The third time around we lose even more, and as more attempts are made, we really get into the small numbers of successful people. The body adapts and as I stated above, goes into "not on my watch" mode and protects itself from the up-to-date eating.

If you are reading this, you know exactly what the diet looks like. You have done it. It worked, then failed you. The modish diet does two things, both detrimental in the long run: it cuts your calories and cuts your carbs or fat too low. This defines all of them. In the back of my book **The Z Diet**, I listed twenty-five of the most popular fad diets at the time it was written and showed how each one of the diets simply had you burn more calories with exercise (and not replace them with food) or cut your calories too low to survive. That is it—that is the secret. Once again, this does work in the short term, but not in the long run or over time.

I could easily spend the next 100 pages discussing all the ins and outs of the modern-day diets, but I am not going to—they are **all** the same, no matter what they claim, or what gimmick they have that others don't, or who has the best-looking celebrity endorsement, or whose exercise program can be done at home in front of your TV, etc. It does not matter. ***On a basic physiologic, metabolic, and hormonal level—they are all the same!***

So, I will use your precious time reading this book to describe the physiologic, metabolic, and hormonal similarities of all the Fat to Fit diets out there.

To further your understanding of a difficult topic (not everyone loves science like I do), I will categorize the common diets into three separate topics of discussion:

1. Hormonal

2. Gastrointestinal (your gut function)

3. Nutritional

## Hormonal

Weight loss, fat loss, muscle loss, muscle gain are all hormone issues. They are not calorie issues, as is obvious by the topic of this book: in the long run, you cannot overexercise or undereat your fat. Period. Calories play a role, the leaner you get (see Appendix I—The Willey Principle), but in the big picture, it's the hormonal changes that occur *with* calorie reduction or increase that matter. That statement would make it arguable that calories have a major role, but if you think of their role as more secondary or in association with fat loss and/or muscle gain, and not directly causative, it will make more sense as you try to discover and understand your body.

Hormones are master controllers. They are messengers on a mission. They work together, in tandem, hand-in-hand, and usually have multiple messages to deliver, depending on their target organ or system. That being said, and contrary to popular belief, to work together, they must all work together—when one is off, they are all off. Think of it as a symphony—when playing together with a good conductor, the music is magical. But let us say the second-string cellist went on a binge the night before and is still suffering from a terrible headache, fuzzy brain, and basically feels terrible. His playing is off, maybe just a little. Maybe so little that a musically naive person in the audience won't hear it. But what about the conductor? He hears it, and he is angry! As he glares at the hung-over cellist missing notes here and there, he starts losing his concentration. Others in the symphony are starting to pick up that sound and the conductor's anger, so they get a little off. Bottom line is, because of that one instrument, the symphony is off. Again—even if the audience does not recognize it, it is tainted—and there will be you know what to pay later. (The analogy here is even if your doctor does not recognize your hormonal chaos, your hormones are in fact off after doing and in some cases while doing a present-day diet—no matter what the labs say on paper).

Another analogy is that of a letter carrier delivering mail. These fine people can be considered messengers, as they have messages to deliver. A message will go from one place to the next on its way to its final destination via the hands of the messengers. Let's say your doctor sends you a simple letter reminding you it is time for a pap smear or prostate exam. Using alcohol as the scapegoat again, let us pretend one of the messengers has been drinking on the job. She loses the letter your doctor sent to you about your favorite exam. Your doctor never hears from you. You miss out on the important exam. Next time you and your doctor visit, he asks, "Why did you not respond to my letter?" assuming up front that you got it, but ignored it. You respond, "What letter?" thinking he never sent you a letter, and he is thinking you just ignored it. This is exactly what happens when you go to your doctor to review a possible hormonal concern. Unless your doctor reviews *all* of the messengers (hormones), controlling for as many variables as possible (time of day, time of month, food, method of detection, etc.), it will be hard to tell when just one is off. You cannot trust the lab value or reference range. You must look at the big picture. The forest through the trees if you will. This is why so many people know they have a thyroid issue, but their doctor says their numbers are fine, so they don't have a thyroid issue. These poor people go on suffering at the advice of their doctor.

The currently suggested eating style messes with hormones. All of them, but in particular the big ones. The lifestyle hormones.

The mother hormones. The bosses. The controllers. The CEO of hormones. The hormones that respond to life. The hormones that respond to food. Go figure—the diets provided to hopeful participants mess up the master hormones—maybe not obvious when you think about it, so let me give you a bit more detail.

When you eat, there is a hormonal response. Your body prepares for the nutrients in several ways, one of them being insulin starting to rise. Insulin is the powerful hormone that takes nutrients out of the blood stream, once digested and absorbed, and deposits them where needed or where the conductor tells it to. This may be your liver, your brain, your muscles, or your fat.

Another hormone that is watching what you are eating is called leptin. The word leptin is derived from the Greek word meaning thin. It is most commonly known as the satiety or fullness hormone, as one of its roles is to tell your brain you have had enough to eat and the storage sites are full. It also senses energy use, and allows the body to utilize fat stores as energy (calorie) sources to keep your body in a preferred (by the body) weight range. Leptin is produced primarily from your fat, in particular subcutaneous (under the skin) fat (some is made in the intestinal tissues), and its job is manifold. It is considered an appetite hormone for one, as when you cut calories or carbs from your diet (i.e., the current diet dogma), leptin decreases. The brain sees this decrease and starts sending signals out to make you eat to bring that mother hormone back up. Those signals are hunger, road rage, grouchiness, and everything else that goes on when the hormones are not happy. These signals, by the way, are partly due to yet another hormone called ghrelin—I call it the road rage hormone, as when it is fired up, people die unless you eat!

Leptin does many things in the body including wound healing and improving our immune system by activating one of the defense army players called T-cells. Hey bodybuilders (or any chronic dieter): how many of you catch a cold as you get ready for a show? Its role in our overall health and function is really incredible, but back to the subject at hand.

Body weight (lean mass and fat mass) regulation is accomplished through precise and effective mechanisms, making it very difficult to lose fat/weight using a calorie sparse diet. As leptin decreases, due to you cutting your carbs and/or calories, hunger increases. As you start to lose body fat producing leptin, your metabolism decreases in an attempt to protect said fat you are trying to get rid of. This makes you hungry. The hungrier you get, the less fat you lose. The hungrier you become, the more likely you are to binge.

Once you binge, you store more fat, as your metabolism has slowed down because your starvation diet had you cut your calories and carbs. You get depressed because your body is not changing the way you had hoped or were expecting, based on the misinformation provided to you by your program, and you cut your calories even more (or exercise harder) and leptin drops even more. Do you see where this is going? A most vicious cycle if there ever was one—one you will never escape.

Leptin's decrease also starts affecting other hormones: thyroid hormone, testosterone, cortisol, your brain hormones, etc. Let me give you a little more detail: remember we discussed above that cortisol increases rT3 and limits the effectiveness of your thyroid hormones? Well leptin does it as well, with a little more kick. In other words, when people come to me and say, "Doctor, I'm gaining weight because my thyroid does not work," I ask them, "Are you dieting?" If they respond in the positive, I quickly advise them they are correct. Due to their dieting, leptin has decreased and their thyroid hormone does not work! This is not something you will find on the lab tests. And, to make matters worse, your accepted program also has you exercising like crazy, as we discussed above. With all this going on, T3 is diminished and this can decrease your ability to absorb nutrients by up to 50%! So, the eating program professed by the popular program has you eating less, causing a hormone issue that causes you to decrease nutrient absorption. Not a good thing. You and your thyroid—0, crazy modern popular diet canon—1. You cannot win this one, sorry.

Testosterone also decreases via the action of leptin. If you consider leptin's role as a lifestyle/mother hormone, it makes sense. Leptin could be considered the gatekeeper of physiologic functions. If your total food intake (calories) is down due to your Fat to Fit eating plan, leptin decreases and tells the rest of your metabolic system to slow down, as well.

Let's say you are a cave man or woman a few thousand years ago, and your food supplies are sparse due to a drought and a poor hunting season. Leptin has decreased in your body, taking testosterone with it. Why? What is one of testosterone's roles? Sex. Sex equals reproduction. Reproduction means kids. Why breed and produce more mouths to feed when there is not enough for you? It's surviv-alistic. Self-preservation. And this self-preservation has a memory. Next time there is a famine, or you decide to do a calorie-restricted diet, your body will remember and go into overdrive to protect your fat stores.

Testosterone also acts as a primary fat burner. It is one of the reasons men have such an easy time losing weight compared to you wonderful women. It is also one of the reasons people take it in the form of anabolic steroids when trying to achieve a look. Your modern diet just made your testosterone tank, you feel horrible, have no libido, no sexual function, you are not building muscle, you are not losing fat—hmm...the thing you are doing to gain that anticipated look is causing the opposite. That makes sense.

There is a very simple and non-scientific way to determine if you have screwed up your leptin kinetics with one (or many) of the programs out there: The "thickness" of your skin, particularly your upper arm or triceps area and possibly thighs. I have seen this quite often in clinical practice and helping people who want that physique. You can see it in any gym, at any time as well—especially in women—thin waists, but thick skin that is only apparent if you grab it. As leptin decreases or you become leptin resistant with the increased exercise and low calories/carbs, the fat starts sticking to the back of arms, legs including calves, upper thighs, etc.—everywhere but the belly!

Again—being very non-scientific here (however I have designed a study to test this so stay tuned), if you are a modern-day diet and exercise program disciple and feel you look relatively lean, especially in the waist/gut region, do the following tests: using some skin fold calipers, have someone pinch the back of your upper arm/triceps area. If your pinch is greater than 15–20 mm, you have some leptin/hormone issues from your program.

## Gastrointestinal (your gut!)

Right now, in the fitness, medical, and lay media, a lot of attention is being focused on the gut. The gut is involved with so many things in the body, from brain health to the immune system; it is truly amazing. One of the common initial contact points for me meeting someone in my clinic who has been following a popular diet and exercise program is gut issues. It is rare to find a healthy gut in a person doing, or having recently done, a well-liked diet and exercise program.

There was a time when getting healthy or lean was just exercises. Now almost all of the modern agendas include an eating plan. This also goes for personal trainers or self-purported fitness experts (who got their degrees from the mirror or admirers of their bodies)—it seems everyone is suddenly a diet and nutrition expert. If you have been in this field as long as I have, you can spot a scam diet from across the room. They are all basically the same. Same food types. Similar macronutrient content. Similar calorie restrictions. They may differ a little in technique (what, when, where, and how often to eat), but from a bird's eye view, they are basically the same. Popular eating plans are not individualized to the person and their needs. This starts to cause havoc in your intestines. It is not always noticeable in the anatomical model of western medicine. In other words, if your guts don't hurt, there is no problem, correct? Nope—incorrect. Many of my clients have gone to a gastroenterologist and paid money to have a camera stuck in each opening of the GI track, only to be told nothing was found.

In a functional model of health and medicine, pain is not the only thing that signals dysfunction. Your get-the-body-you-want diet adversely affects your gut and may show up as depression, lack of energy, or joint and body aches, not just a case of the runs! Which, of course, affects every other aspect of your life and eventually leads to failure of the program itself.

When your gut starts to get wrecked from the chic diet pro-gram, many things occur: low to poor microbiome (gut bacteria), also called dysbiosis, food intolerances, and inflammation. These tend to build on each other, as the more bacterial disruptions, the more food intolerances, the more inflammation, the more you get of the same. A very vicious cycle. Then all the sequela of said gut issues—every medical problem you can think of! This list would include: depression, joint issues, asthma, brain fog, memory issues, muscle aches and pains, skin changes, including acne and other rashes, autoimmune diseases, heart palpitations—when your gut does not work well, you get yourself in trouble. If anything on this list raises your eyebrows, your gut needs some help. Of course, there are several other variables, but the gut is involved with all of them, and a healthy gut is of utmost importance for overall health.

A healthy gut can be defined as you having the following:
- More than one bowel movement a day
- Feeling good and energized after eating
- No undigested food in the stools
- No extreme food or drink cravings
- Balanced moods
- Good sleep and tons of energy upon awakening

Signs of a gut negatively influenced by a modern diet and exercise program include:
- Less than one bowel movement a day
- Feeling fatigued and weak after eating

- Indigestion after food intake
- Producing a lot of gas (from either end)
- Food cravings
- Mood disorders
- Poor sleep and waking up fatigued

This poor gut health can also cause direct gut symptoms such as excessive gas, nausea, bloating, heartburn, and abdominal pain and/or distention.

Your gut uses 1/3 of the blood flow from your heart and demands a large percentage of your overall metabolism. Much of your immune system surrounds the gut, with over 80% of the lymph nodes in the body neighboring it. That means your immune system (analogous to a military) knows where to anticipate foreign invaders coming into your body—through your gut! When the gut breaks down, due to a vigorous diet and exercise program, a vicious cycle of feeling rotten starts to occur and all those conditions I mentioned a few paragraphs ago can start to show up.

One of the reasons a modern diet program survivor has gut issues is because the eating plan does not meet nutritional needs. With the high cortisol levels, gut function and gut bacteria are changed. Mal-digestion begins and causes additive changes in the gut microbiome or gut bacteria. At the same time, the hormonal changes and the overexercising (discussed above) and the nutritional deficiencies (described below), all add to the problem.

Changes in the gut microbiome or gut bacteria are called dysbiosis, or an imbalance of the gut bacteria. The lining of your gut is also very sensitive to your nutritional and lifestyle choices. The lining is replaced every week or so and, if you are in a high-stress environment with poor nutrient intake, the gut lining fails to adequately support itself and do its job. In addition, when following a Fat to Fit program, one tends to do a lot of things that can be very detrimental to the gut: increase in free radical generation, frequent and many times overdone use of anti-inflammatory drugs or NSAIDS, such as Ibuprofen, Aspirin, Aleve, etc., due to all the soreness one encounters doing the program—these things damage the gut.

Dysbiosis associated with a Fat to Fit program causes the loss of good bacteria and that situation allows for bad bacteria and other species (such as yeast) to overgrow and take over. It also changes the way vitamins and cofactors are produced. Your ability to detoxify is also hampered by poor gut health. These all can lead to what has been termed a "leaky gut." A leaky gut is loss of the good bacteria and lining of the intestines, leading to increased permeability. Increased permeability allows toxins to get in, as well as larger proteins that would not normally be allowed to cross the gut barrier. This can stimulate the immune system to react and is the basic set up for autoimmune diseases.

Fixing the gut is essential and I will get into the proper gut testing in Chapter 8 under Bowel Bollix. Adding the proper pre- and probiotic is crucial, but you really should be tested to see which ones you need and then plan to rotate the probiotics on a regular basis. Taking the same probiotic for months (years) at a time can cause that particular strain of bacteria to overgrow and take over (ultimate power = ultimate corruption). I think the best way to get good probiotics in your system is to make them with homemade yogurt, kombucha, etc., not via a pill. If you do take the probiotic pills, get the ones kept in the refrigerator at your favorite health food store, and be sure to use them within one month (i.e., only purchase one month's fill at a time, as they tend to die easily). Prebiotics, or the probiotic food, can be found in any form of fiber. The concern here is if you have a crappy gut (snicker) or irritable bowel, eating fiber is hard to do, as it just makes things worse. Adding a tablespoon of fermented foods, such as sauerkraut or kimchi, once or twice a day tends to be a little easier on your gut in this situation. Good gut bacteria ferment resistant starch and fiber to produce short chain fatty acids (SCFA) such as n-butyrate, which is the fuel source for the cells of your colon. Low levels of this fuel are analogous to trying to drive your car without gas—it does not work well. There are supplements available that act as good prebiotics, as well as supplements that contain the SCFA to help get your gut working again.

Understanding how a prevalent diet and exercise program damages the gut is essential to your overall ability to heal from the program. As I mentioned in the first paragraph of this section, there is a lot of emphasis on the gut right now in all forms of media, but you need to fix stress and cortisol levels **BEFORE** the gut is fixed. This, of course, means fixing problem #1, as discussed above, as too much exercise is an enormous stress on the body and therefore affects the gut.

A quick lead-in to **Problem #3—The Supplements and the Drugs**. A number of these chemicals disrupt gut function and bacteria with the power and effectiveness of antibiotics. That is something I do not believe has been mentioned in any study, blog, or forum concerning these drugs. It is something which also must be considered, as you come to understand the pathophysiology and dangers of current diet and exercise thinking.

## Nutrients

Low calorie eating, like most diet programs out there profess, is a strong influencing factor in vitamin and mineral deficiency. Add the intense training as we discussed above, and it is almost guaranteed you are lacking some vital cofactors in your body! Many programs have you take some vitamins during your torture time; however, there are studies that show that in this low calorie/high exercise situation, even with supplementation, the deficiencies are still present.

Unless you are on a very good, tailored program that individualizes your nutrient needs, based on lab work from your very own body, you are nutrient deprived and depleted doing a modern diet and exercise program.

Trending eating plans tend to be low in a lot of important nutrients. To name but a few: B vitamins, magnesium, calcium, potassium, fat-soluble vitamins such as vitamin D, E, A, and K, and many of the more obscure (yet very important) amino acids such as taurine. A few of the programs suggest supplementing vitamins and minerals, but the majority do not, due to fears of lawsuits and likely the knowledge that supplementation protocols really need personalization.

Many of the diet and exercise programs that remove fat or carbs from your table allow for all sorts of issues over time. Fat is an essen-tial nutrient. It is involved in absorption of fat-soluble vitamins, energy production, and protection of lipid membranes in all your cells. All of this starts to decline when you remove fat from your diet. Carbohydrates are not essential for life, but they are essential for the type of exercise that so many widespread programs suggest. You simply cannot completely remove a macronutrient from your diet and do well.

The extreme exercise depletes minerals, in particular, magnesium (Mg+). Magnesium is responsible for over 300 metabolic functions in the body, including but not limited to: production of ATP, brain and nerve function, balance of other electrolytes such as sodium and potassium, blood sugar metabolism, muscle (including your heart) function, bone strength, and oxygen uptake. When this essential mineral gets low, you get muscle tightness and your propensity for injury skyrockets. Of course, you blame yourself for a faulty movement while exercising or something, but in reality, it can be a very dangerous deficiency and the cause of your injuries. Magnesium deficiency causes you to get easily fatigued, not only in the gym but all day. To the point that Monster drinks and coffee just do not seem to work like they used to. Your stamina disappears. You become a "Nervous Nelly," even though you have never had problems with anxiety in the past.

A low level or imbalance of amino acids causes all sorts of issues. In your body there are 40,000 different proteins made up from the different amino acids. They are involved in detoxification, making neurotransmitters (brain hormones), and just about every physiological function in the body. When you start to get deficient on an up-to-date diet and exercise program, symptoms such as fatigue, allergies, emotional problems, depression, anxiety, headaches, and frequent infections are commonplace. Your blood sugars and lipids go screwy, and your sleep becomes much less than required. I could cover each one and what happens to you when you become deficient but suffice it to say—it ain't good!

This is one area people will argue with, as it is claimed that these programs equate to good eating. That is true if you are comparing the diet of someone who eats McDonald's for breakfast, Wendy's for lunch, and then drinks a six pack and eats two bags of Doritos© every night. But when you put it in perspective, the lower amounts, the monotony of foods, the vigorous exercise, and the stress inherent in each fashionable program—you have nutrient deficiencies! Even the high protein diets in a few of the suggested programs do not account for individual need(s). Protein requirements are very individualized, and it cannot be understated that a "suggested" amount (which is always too low as these programs cut your calories too low; therefore, your nutrients are too low) is never enough to maintain health and longevity for your body while doing the program.

The crazy diet and exercise program also ruins the gut mucosa (lining of the gut tube) causing a change in your ability to absorb nutrients. This is due to the fact that the chronic stress involved in the program keeps the sympathetic nervous system at a high "tone" and thereby limits the ability of the vagus nerve to protect the gut mucosal membrane.

Nutrient deficiencies can also be caused by a few of the drugs and even a few supplements people use when following a number of these popular programs. These depleted nutrients include the B vitamins, zinc, minerals such as calcium, magnesium, potassium, fat-soluble vitamins, CoQ10, and many others depending on the drugs or supplements being used. Speaking of supplements, this paragraph also allows me a nice flow to the next section of the book.

# CHAPTER 6
## Problem 3–The Supplements and the Drugs

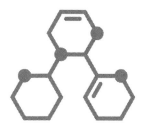

Many modern diet and exercise programs suggest supplements. A lot of current trainers and gym rats suggest drugs. Neither is necessarily independently dangerous or at fault; they are just additive to the inborn error of the trendy program. Bodybuilders and fitness competitors have managed to find a short-term "fix" to the problems that occur with the low calories and vigorous exercise by using drugs. Anabolic/androgenic steroids (AAS) to combat the low androgens (like testosterone) that occur with an intense program, thyroid medications for crumbling thyroids, amphetamines (speed—both legal and illegal) for the lack of energy and terrible hunger issues, etc.

In this section of the book, I am neither condemning nor condoning the supplements and drugs I will refer to. I am simply showing you how they are part of the problem with the current diet and exercise mentality. I think supplements and drugs, the right ones (also being the legal ones) certainly have a place in a recovery program. I will cover a few of them in the *RecoverMe* section of this book, but until then—let's discuss a few of the more common and popular supplements and drugs.

## The Supplements

Ahh, the supplements. There are far too many to mention, so I won't—I will mention categories and a few of the general ones in use but, most important, I will discuss how these supplements add to the problems of the modern diet and exercise programs.

Supplement, as the word implies, is the amount by which an angle is less than 180 degrees…*wait…that's in geometry*. The definition of a supplement is something that completes or enhances something else when added to it. The FDA's definition is:

A dietary supplement is a product intended for ingestion that contains a "dietary ingredient" intended to add further nutritional value to (supplement) the diet. A "dietary ingredient" may be one, or any combination, of the following substances:

- a vitamin
- a mineral
- an herb or other botanical
- an amino acid
- a dietary substance for use by people to supplement the diet by increasing the total dietary intake
- a concentrate, metabolite, constituent, or extract

Dietary supplements may be found in many forms, such as tablets, capsules, soft gels, gel caps, liquids, or powders. Some dietary supplements can help ensure that you get an adequate dietary intake of essential nutrients; others may help you reduce your risk of disease, and so on.

## Nutritional Substitutions

Several of the suggested supplements in most modern popular diet and exercise programs are to cover up for nutritional deficiencies. That's not a bad thing by any means, but it should pull into question the eating plans suggested within the programs. These supplements would include amino acids, multivitamins, protein powders, meals, bars, chips, etc. They also include several supplements that can be of great benefit in certain conditions/situations—such as conditions caused by the diet and exercise program itself.

The problem arises when so many processed meal replacements and their accompanying supplements take over for real food. In my clinical practice, I have people fill out food diaries to get a handle on what is crossing their lips. On many occasions, my patient's list is nothing more than processed foods such as protein shakes, meal replacement bars, and a handful of supplements. Not only do we start to see problems with all the chemicals involved, but we also see concerns due to the lack of real food.

God-made food such as fruits and vegetables, organic meats, nuts and seeds and occasionally dairy, etc. contain a far wider variety of naturally occurring vitamins and minerals than what you can find in a capsule, powder, or meal replacement. Antioxidants, phytonutrients, and the fiber found in fresh raw fruits and vegetables, for example, work together in combination to provide a greater nutritional benefits than supplements or artificial foods could ever do.

## Thermogenics, Energy Supplements, Appetite Suppressants

Thermogenics, energy supplements, and appetite suppressants are all classified together as they all work on hormones in the brain and body responsible for just that: heat producing, energy providing, and appetite suppression. A huge number of supplements in currently suggested programs are used to decrease appetite and/or increase energy. Again—not necessarily a bad thing, but often (if not all of the time for those willing to use them) these become **THE** way people maintain function outside of their exercise setting. Take a thermogenic or energy supplement to exercise. Use one a few hours later to curb your appetite. Use more mid-afternoon, as you are dragging and mentally a space cadet, etc. Eventually, it becomes impossible to function in your place of work, home with the kids, out with the spouse, etc. without them. This should tell you that the fuel tank is low, and you need to pull over and get some gas. Running on fumes (fumes being these supplements in this case) certainly applies here.

Eventually, due either to constant panic attacks and anxiety, lack of sleep as you took your last one too late in the day, a heart rate beating out of your chest (as they all increase heart rate and blood pressure), or you quit the suggested diet and exercise program—you quit taking the supplements. Then everything really crumbles.

These supplements/drugs keep you awake and energized, keep your hunger down, and allow mental focus because they modify brain hormones responsible for doing just that. Over time, these hormones start to deplete especially because your protein require-ments are not being met as these brain hormones are derived from amino acids found in your diet.

Yes, your body can make new ones, but your body also literally becomes dependent on the supplements to kick-start the hormones. When you stop taking them for any of the reasons mentioned above, you crash—and crash hard. Crashing hard causes binging and your body begging for foods that will provide quick relief from the way you feel—that would be high sugar, high fat, highly-processed foods that spike insulin (that causes fat gain) and increase brain hormones, such as serotonin for a quick, but short-lived relief from said crash.

Remember what you learned on Sesame Street and from your preschool teacher? What goes up must come down.

You start to gain fat and lose that awesome physique you just worked so hard for, so you go back to the heavy, hard exercise and start deteriorating even more.

## Prohormones and Other "Undescribed/Unclassified" Supplements

These likely should be under the drug section below, but since you can purchase most of these over the counter, I will cover a few of them here.

A prohormone is a precursor of a hormone, such as a peptide, that is cleaved to create a shorter polypeptide hormone or a hormone that is made active by peripheral metabolism. The FDA came down on these a few years ago, stating, in short, they were drugs and, therefore, could not be sold over the counter. However, as with any performance enhancing or mind-altering drug, the "bathtub chemists" are way ahead of the law and ability to test these products. A whole new generation of prohormones and other drugs continue to show up. Many of them have very good and notable effects/benefits, and since they are sold in a legal way, over the counter, the impression created is that they are safe, without side effects or future concerns. This makes both men and women basically feel good and safe about their steroid use.

Unfortunately, taking them is not without negative side effects. Many of them acting as a substrate to hormones downstream, wind up turning off natural hormone production. When the user stops the prohormone, most with the goal to increase androgens (testosterone being the best-known androgen), all of their own hormones downstream have been dampened and users go without any hormones for some time—until the body recovers, if ever. With the added stress of the diet and exercise of a currently suggested or popular program, and now lacking a few key hormones responsible for everything from energy, sex drive, muscle building, fat losing, etc., the crash is incredibly common. In other words, these supplements/drugs that helped you get your physique are part of the reason you lose your fine-tuned body so quickly after you stop the program.

One quick comment not related to the book's topic: I have seen organ issues, such as liver and kidney failure, with these supplements/drugs. Young people taking them may wind up in the Intensive Care Unit due to bad problems that are eventually narrowed down to these supplements/drugs. That is playing with fire, in my opinion. All the potential side effects of these supplements/drugs are beyond the scope of this book. Just be aware of other, not often reported concerns with these chemicals.

A few of the go-getter programs and trainers suggest peptides such as Sermorelin, GRP-6, GRP-2, etc. that increase growth hormone. These peptides, simplistically put, cause an increase in one's own production of growth hormone and IGF-1 (insulin growth fac-tor 1—the major "actor" for growth hormone). Growth hormone, some would claim, is the fountain of youth enabling the body to burn more fat and increase muscle mass/size. While that is true and potentially of great benefit, the cost is something few can maintain for long periods of time. When the supplements/drugs are stopped, with everything else going awry with the diet and exercise program, it feeds into the dysfunction of the underlying Fat to Fit concern.

SARMs (selective androgen receptor modulators) are made to attach to the androgen receptor without causing any of the negative problems seen with anabolic/androgenic steroids (AAS). They work by altering gene expression by binding at the androgen receptors of muscles. This is very beneficial, if true, as muscles could grow without a lot of the side effects of AAS, including virilization in women. This means that development of masculine traits, found in men, might not be generated in women when SARMs are used. These include but are not limited to: body hair (guys, can you imagine being with a girl with a hairy chest and back??), voice changes (deepening like a man's), and clitoral enlargement. Yes, you heard that right. Clitorises that look like little penises are very common in women who use AAS! As this is a PG-rated book, I will not go into what I have seen.

The thought and intention are good, but not enough is known about these drugs to make a final determination as to their safety. For now, we need to consider that these drugs can eventually cause hormone issues like those as described with the prohormones.

As I said before, there are literally hundreds of supplements I could cover, but the goal of this book is to present the problem, touch on a few reasons the problem exists, and provide you with a solution, so this will not be an exhaustive supplement review.

## Drugs

Admittedly, in the big picture among the millions of people who do any one of the modern diet and exercise programs, drugs are only used by a small percentage. That being said, the percentage is increasing daily, as the availability of these drugs on the Internet and the extreme desire of people to obtain that desired image at any cost are also increasing rapidly. I am going to cover five drugs I see being used most commonly from middle school children (yes, kids!) to men and women in their 70s. These five drugs are examples of many other drugs that fit into their respective categories, so please we aware that there are many others.

## Oxandrolone–Anavar®

Oxandrolone, under the original trade name Anavar, is an anabolic/androgenic steroid (AAS). It is more anabolic (promotes positive nitrogen retention, muscle growth, fat burning and all the sought-after benefits of AAS) than its androgenic (relating to the development of male characteristics including body hair, loss of hair on the head, change/growth of the male genital organs and mass). Therefore, it is likely the most popular AAS in women, as the androgenic side effects are "lessened" (notice I did not say absent).

The AAS users and underground consider it a "cutting drug," as it aids the user in leaning up—losing fat while maintaining muscle mass.

I am convinced that oxandrolone is in the water supply of several of the gyms I have been to, as the number of lean and muscular women out there is really hard to believe. Twenty years ago, it was so rare to see what is now seen daily in the gyms and oxandrolone is one of the reasons. It is an oral steroid, making it popular as it does not involve needles, and it is likely one of the only steroids out there that directly increases fat loss. It has legitimate medical purposes, including preventing weight loss in really sick people, increasing blood counts in severe anemics, treating the muscle wasting caused by drugs such as prednisone, and protecting bone in osteoporosis, to name a few.

The modern diet and exercise issue? You cannot maintain that look unless oxandrolone is taken continuously. In other words, stop the drug, lose the look. Something many people have chosen to do in trade for long-term consequences. No matter how safe something is assumed to be, everything has consequences.

The majority of people who use oxandrolone use it for contest prep or show prep, they eventually come off the drug (after the show) that helped them gain that amazing look they were after.

Add that to the other problems discussed with the modern diet and exercise mentality or more the better, and all the issues are exemplified a hundred-fold. It also makes it very difficult for those wanting to obtain that look, but do not take the drug. They never get that look their trainer has or the girl who keeps winning shows and they cut their calories farther, and exercise harder, only adding to the concern. Do you see the problem? The drug affects everyone around it, taking it or not.

## Clenbuterol–"Clen"

Clen increases your energy to the point you appear to have attention deficit disorder, burns fat like a furnace, and builds (or at the very least protects) lean mass while you are on the extreme diet and exercise program. Pretty much the perfect drug if not for the side effects and what happens to your body when you stop taking it.

Clenbuterol is a non-FDA approved drug used to treat asthma in other countries of the world. It is not approved, or used in America, as the powers-that-be feel its risks outweigh its benefits and with drugs like Albuterol for asthma, it is not used here.

Clenbuterol is what we in the medical field call a beta-agonist. It is a stimulant. It "stimulates" the beta receptors on various cells. Also called a sympathomimetic, or a drug that works on the sympathetic nervous system, it increases the release of norepinephrine and epinephrine. Stimulation of beta receptors in the lungs causes the lung tubes (bronchials) to dilate or get bigger for more air flow. This is done via the beta 2 receptors. It excites the heart to increase its rate by stimulating the beta 1 receptors. At the level of the "powerhouses of the cells," the mitochondria, it stimulates beta 2 receptors and increases heat production or metabolism. In the fat or adipose tissue, it stimulates beta 3 receptors, causing an increase in lipolysis or the release of fat for energy. Beta 3 receptors also increase thermogenesis, increase heat production in the muscles. The beta 2 and 3 receptors are what those desiring extreme leanness are after.

As a stimulant, it causes increased energy and a sense of well-being. If you can deal with the increased heart rate, anxiety, and sweating—you feel pretty good taking this drug.

It has been proposed that it increases lean mass (in laboratory animals), but this effect in humans appears to be minimal, if present at all. It could be argued that, at the very least, it protects lean mass, while on a low-calorie diet, but that may be a stretch as well.

It is not used as a weight loss drug in everyone as its benefits are more noticeable if you are already lean. Hence, the popularity with physique artists such as bodybuilders and fitness competitors.

The side effects are few but quite noticeable. I have clocked a few users' heart rates at 190 while at rest. Constant sweat pouring off brows and a nervous anxiety that could only be equaled by meth are but a few. Reporting to the emergency room or a doctor's office with chest pain is also very common. We see it more often than one would think in the urgent cares I own in my small town. Case reports of cardiac arrhythmia are also out there.

Those are all important to note, and many people are happy to live with said side effects as their focus on the body goal is far more powerful. So back to the intent of this book: what happens when you stop the drug and everything it was masking becomes apparent?

As you likely anticipated, there is a crash. A brain crash, as your neurotransmitters have been fried by the drug and you can't remember anything anymore. An emotional crash, as you turn in to a raging lunatic or cry at every turn for the same brain chemicals disarray as I mentioned above. And finally, a fat crash—crash in this case being a large rebound back up and fat gain as never before!

The drug is usually stopped at the same time the crazy diet and exercise program is stopped, so you, by now, can anticipate the effects on the once beautiful and shapely physique.

## Phentermine-Adipex, Fastin, Lomaira, etc.

Phentermine is a schedule IV appetite suppressant that has been around since the 1950s. It is a safe drug in terms of known or common side effects associated with this type of drug. It is also a sympathomimetic, or a drug that works on the sympathetic nervous system. There is a transient elevation of blood pressure when one takes it, but that only lasts a few days. It can make you anxious, a bit jittery/nervous, and speed up your heart rate ( nothing like

Clen, however). It has a few cousins that have a lot more side effects, including the possibility of addiction, but those are less well known, and they are a bit more controlled, being schedule III drugs.

The danger with this drug in a modern diet and exercise program is that it allows you to ignore, or possibly not even realize, your body's need for nourishment. Thus, it can perpetuate the downward spiral of a state-of-the-art diet and exercise program. It also provides some energy, running on fumes as I mentioned above, so your body's overall stress level and deterioration on the diet and exercise program are accentuated.

I see doctors prescribe Phentermine all the time for the depression that accompanies excessive exercise and restrictive dieting. The depletion of brain chemicals caused by the currently suggested diet and exercise program is greatly accentuated with this drug. That is not good.

As the other drugs mentioned in this section, once you stop taking it, your crash changes from a 15-mph fender bender to an 80-mph head-on collision. The rebound from it is tremendous, especially the mental/emotional rebound. Even if you were to maintain your program, stopping this drug would cause you some issues, including unwanted fat gain, which furthers your attempts to lose it—that is, you decrease your calories more and increase your exercise. Back to our vicious cycle.

## T3 or Triiodothyronine

Triiodothyronine or T3 is a thyroid hormone involved in almost every metabolic action in the body. From basal metabolic rate, heart rate, body temperature, and heat production, there are only a few tissues/organs in the body not affected by this hormone (your spleen for example, but that has never been much of a helper in physique development). For the popular diet and exercise program disciple, the increase in body oxygen and energy consumption is what they are after.

To understand some of the potential concern with this drug, I need to provide you with some basic understanding of these hormones—Thyroid Hormones 101, if you will.

Thyroxine and triiodothyronine, T4 and T3 respectively, are produced in the thyroid. They are stimulated, or produced, in response to thyroid-stimulating hormone (TSH) from your pituitary gland in your head. They work on a feedback mechanism. A negative feedback mechanism to be precise, meaning that, as the level of thyroid hormones goes up (directly from the thyroid or from taking thyroid medication), the TSH goes down. If there is not enough thyroid medication in the body, TSH will go up, as if to yell at the thyroid to get to work. The more the body needs T4 and T3, the "louder" or higher TSH will go.

In the body, T4 can be considered the precursor to T3—in other words, your body converts T4 (having four iodines attached to the molecule) to T3 (having three iodines attached to the molecule after the removal of one by some enzymes called deiodinases). T3 is roughly four times more powerful than T4 and, therefore, it is considered the "active" hormone.

When one takes thyroid hormones, this negative feedback mechanism works very well. You take T3, and your TSH drops, so as to be quiet and not ask the thyroid for any T4 or T3.

I mentioned it in the section on eating under the auspices of a modern diet and exercise program, but it needs emphasized or at the least restated. When a patient comes to me or any/all doctors out there with the complaint of an inability to lose weight, whether they mention it or not (and a large number mention it) this is what is stated, "Doctor, I am convinced I cannot lose weight because my thyroid does not work." If they are dieting, they are correct. Extremes of caloric restriction change the way T3 works in the body. It's the body's way of slowing things down, as the energy supply is scarce.

T3 being a hormone that increases oxygen and energy consumption (i.e., burns calories) is limited as the body tries to protect itself from the starvation. That is why taking thyroid hormones seems to be of such great benefit while dieting, as they increase energy consumption. I am also convinced that extremes of diet and exercise destroy the metabolism following the diet via this protective mechanism. And it appears from examples and studies done on the good people who diet like this (such as "The Biggest Loser" contestants) that the damage takes a really long time, and the right program, to heal. It never fixes itself, and that is one of the reasons people gain their weight back so quickly and then can never lose it again.

Many Fat to Fit program users, especially the physique artists, turn to this hormone/drug to counter the natural decrease in metabolism caused by the program itself. While that makes sense, what do they do next?

If they decide to keep taking the T3, they change the way the body and thyroid function. Taking T3 suppresses thyroid-stimulating hormone (TSH). As I mentioned before, TSH is released from the pituitary gland in the brain to tell the thyroid to release the thy-roid hormones T3 and T4. When T3 is taken, the thyroid stops pro-ducing and the body suffers, as T4 is also needed, particularly by the brain. T3 is the active hormone, as I mentioned. However, it cannot find its way to the brain to do its essential work there, as it cannot cross the blood brain barrier (BBB). T4 is needed, as it *does* cross the BBB and the brain tissues then convert T4 to T3 to do its work in the brain. Without T4, there are problems including fatigue, depression, poor sleep, failed memory, etc.

If the T3 user decides to stop the T3, it takes a while for the body to recover normal thyroid function in a time when it is so very needed—following the overexercising and undereating program. Hence, the additive effect/problem this particular drug adds to the users. The overexercising and undereating both directly and indirectly wrecks hormones, and the participant of the program uses hormones to counter act the effects of said program. At the end of it, everything is out of whack and a terrible downward spiral is created.

## Testosterone

Testosterone has been a very out-front topic over the last few years. It is as popular as both hated and loved, depending on who you talk to. There is a ton of information out there, including a book I wrote on the topic called **The T Club**. I won't go into a lot of detail here other than to discuss how it is utilized in a modern diet and exercise program.

Both men and women utilize testosterone for fitness/body goals. With the general acceptance of the "low T" state as a medical diagnosis, both men and women are using it under legal pretense by getting their doctors involved. A low T level is found on a lab test, and the person is prescribed testosterone in one form or another. All fine and dandy and certainly in several cases, perfectly legitimate. But as you have learned, the modern suggestion of overexercising and undereating in and of itself can cause low T. If it is replaced under this condition, it will worsen the eventual problem.

When testosterone is replaced, in particular by injections or pellet therapy, levels climb high quickly. This is very comparable to methamphetamine—the first time someone uses it, they feel really good. It is also comparable to methamphetamine, as one finds it very hard to get the same high again with continued use.

Testosterone with inappropriate dosing changes the gut, causes weight gain and bloating, and sets people, particularly women, up for further failure. The longer they replace it, the less it seems to work. It changes the hormonal cascade that is so important for optimal health. Exogenous (from the outside) use turns off the inside production, causing more problems for the user, as in a lot of instances, they stop using it when they stop the program. Like the thyroid discussed above, this causes a number of concerns. The hormone cascade is in disarray when you need it most.

In summary of the supplement/drug section, I must mention something that can be taken for granted when one is standing in the trees and fails to see the forest and that is the financial burden of all the supplements and drugs. I honestly have witnessed divorces, fights, houses being lost, and other financial strain (that just adds to the stress of the modern diet and exercise program), when the goal to get that body exceeds common sense and responsibility. I am continually amazed at how much money tends to be spent on these types of programs. Even if you have money to burn, it's a burden. Lifestyle and recovery programs, like I will soon describe, do cost money, but they are usually front-loaded (to make the correct diagnosis and get the initial treatment going). Real life and livable lifestyle programs do not come with the financial burden of a modern and popular diet and exercise program, and that, in and of itself, is healing.

# CHAPTER 7

# Diets Written Under the Guise of Medical Supervision

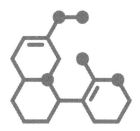

This is a totally different array of eating plans, as they have the appearance of being healthy because they are provided by medical clinics. These are doctor diets or very low calorie supplemental diets that fall into the Fat to Fit categories. In dietetic terminology In dietetic terminology, they are called very low-calorie diets, VLCD, or very low energy diets, VLED. I like the second option, as low energy is exactly what you get from them. New Direction, Optifast, Medifast, and the hCG diet are a few of the more popular ones. Entire medical conferences and medical societies profess these eating plans, as they do cause weight loss. Put anyone on an 800-calorie liquid or supplement diet, and they will lose weight, at least the first time they try it. These diets are controversial due to safety issues and long-term efficacy, as caloric intake is far below the basal metabolic rate of virtually all adults.

VLED are also called protein sparing modified fasts. Calories in these diets are in the range 400–800 per day. The amount of protein, when calculated out, is 1.5 grams per kilogram of ideal body weight for males, and 1.2 grams per kilogram for females (typically 75–105 grams per day). Carbohydrates are usually around 50–100 grams per day to minimize nitrogen loss (muscle loss) and lessen the chance of people getting into ketosis. Fat in the diet is around 10–20 grams a day, emphasizing essential fatty acids.

Companies that make the meals, shakes, cookies, and protein bars for these diets fortify them with nutrients you will miss due to the low caloric amounts and processing. These would include: potassium, calcium, sodium, vitamins, and mineral supplementation of at least Recommended Daily Allowance (RDA), fiber, etc.

Safety is emphasized in these eating plans, hence the doctor involvement. The emphasis from the companies that make this type of diet (listed above) claim these scale weight reducing diets must be nutritionally adequate except for their energy (calorie) content. They claim these diets minimize excessive losses of body protein as excessive weight (in the obese), on average, is 75% fat and 25% fat-free mass.

While it is most certainly true that loss of lean body mass must be minimized, it is very difficult with this type of eating plan. I know—I measure body composition on everyone, not just scale weight. If you think about it, it becomes obvious: Lean body mass contains only 363 kcal per pound. In other words, (and simplified), muscle is 20% protein, 80% water. When you remove an extreme number of calories from your diet, you will lose lean body mass or muscle. Some of these diets target lean body mass, so it looks like they are really working—that would be the 20 pounds in 10-day diet or any diet that claims rapid and quick weight loss. Yes, a lot of the scale weight is water, but the muscles are not immune to the diets effects.

If one of these very popular diets decreases your calories by 1,000 a day, you could theoretically lose 2 ¾ pounds per day! While this might fulfill your wildest diet dreams, you will pay for it later. Quality weight loss must be paced!

If these diets are not formulated appropriately, they may result in generalized protein depletion, followed by myocardial intracellular protein depletion. Those are fancy words for bad things happening to your heart, such as ventricular arrhythmias!

Weight loss by these diet supporter's definition, is a decrease in scale weight in a short period of time—30 to 60 days on average. What they don't tell you is that it is a Fat to Fit to Fat program and your weight **will** come back eventually. It is impossible to stay on the supplements and suggested calories forever. Your metabolism, energy, and sense of well-being all slow down to meet that low caloric intake and you will eventually fail. The weight comes back and comes back with a vengeance, as I have described above.

Since we are a "fix me now" society, wanting to see quick results to keep us motivated, these diets are perfect for our impatient con-sumer mentality. Add in the fact that a weight loss specialist/doctor is telling you to do the diet, and it must be safe, effective, and work well—right?

The reason they are professed by certain medical professionals and societies is because, before companies such as those listed above started supplying the supplements that contained fortified nutrients, participating in an extreme diet like this could kill you. In the 1970s and early 1980s, there were case reports of extreme weight loss using these types of programs and the people following them dropping like flies because of cardiac (heart) arrhythmias due to electrolyte deficiencies, etc. Today, they are nutrient fortified, so that is less likely to happen, as I mentioned above.

Side effects for these processed, fake (but fortified) meals/diets include: gut distress such as diarrhea, fatigue, mineral loss, cold intolerance, gout, sagging skin, libido changes, anemia, brittle nails, hair loss, amenorrhea (your periods stop girls), insomnia, depression, gallstones (up to 25% of users!), anxiety, muscle cramps, etc.

They have some direct contraindications including: diabetes, pregnancy, lactation (breast feeding), older than the young age of 65, or younger than 16, a history of heart disease, a history of seizure disorders, if you use a lot of ibuprofen, or are on any number of medications. Also of concern are those with high risk occupations, as you could get dizzy and fall to your death or run over someone while driving.

Doctors sell them from their offices for profit, and do a full workup on potential users, including basic labs and chemistries, EKGs to check the heart, etc. It is a good business model if you are in it for business, but unless the basic physiology and nature of the program is understood, it is a scam. No one keeps the weight off forever without proper support and hormonal retribution.

Companies that make these diets have doctors distribute them as doctors can make the absolute misery of only taking in 800 calories a day, in artificial form and having to stay away from your favorite foods, a little more tolerable. That is done via the power of the prescription pad! Appetite suppressants, mood elevators, opioid antagonists, etc. all can make the month or two your scale weight decreases seem a little better. But, like all good things, it must come to an end. And then the Piper needs to be paid.

I have already stated all the reasons these diets don't work in the long term—the hormonal changes, the stress on the body causing high cortisol levels, and the body's incredible defense system that kicks in and goes into "save all the fat you can" when you go off the diet.

That being said, *they have a place when done correctly*. With the proper hormonal support and understanding of fixing the underlying issue at hand, medically supervised diets could be a quick starting point if the follow up is appropriate. They also have a place in medicine for quick weight loss needed for an urgent (not emergent) surgery, for example.

Again, the issue comes back to wanting it right now, and not being patient enough to get the fat off correctly, thereby setting yourself up for failure, due to the basic pathophysiology inherited in modern diet and exercise programs.

# PART III – THE FIX

## How to Be Your Best, Feel Your Best, and Look Your Best... for Life!

Do you know any sumo wrestlers? These are fat AND fit people.

They exercise like crazy, making their visceral fat or fat around the gut minimal. Research goes back and forth on this, but it is felt that this makes them healthy as defined by minimal heart issues, fewer blood pressure issues, insulin issues, etc., as visceral fat is linked to these problems. Their hormone-producing power fat under their skin, however, is abundant. This is the subcutaneous fat that produces leptin, something I will dive into in more detail below. These large men have several hormone issues, like any modern exercise and diet program survivor, even though they "look" completely different. I have had some success with a few of my patients when I compare them to a sumo wrestler (after they punch me in the nose, let the thought settle in, then get the point). The body does what it has to as survival is its job. The job of your body from the neck down is to protect the neck up!

To fix this problem caused by modern dieting and exercise programs, it may be of benefit to you to always think your body has a mind of its own and is out to protect you. Once you tell yourself you are a thin, muscular, amazing looking person after following a torturous program, your body will decide otherwise and you will likely lose it. It's the truth! If you are reading this book looking for a way out, you already know it.

The 5% of people who actually make up 100% of the "body I want" pictures out there in all the different social media platforms' motivational boards, will tell you that you just have to think positive and you can look just like them. No, you must be realistic about your own goal. Not all of us can look like those blessed 5%, airbrushed and all. Nor should we want to. If you happened to ask how they felt (quality of life question) and they honestly answered, a large percentage of them would summarize it in two words: awful. The crazy diet and exercise program that got them there will ask for reparation very soon.

If you are fat and, if you want to fix it, accept it and make a change. First, accept who you are and fight to feel good. Let your body goals take a back seat to quality of life. In my 30+ years of helping people get the bodies they want, those that do the best feel good first.

I have nothing against a good motivational post or picture, but this book is about real life. Sadness, anger, and grief are emotions just like happiness and joy. They are OK. Let me teach you how to be the best *you* you can be. Start by accepting yourself, accepting your body, and shoot for a great quality of life!

## *RecoverMe*

You are finally at the meat of the book, likely what you have been waiting for, so thank you for sticking with me up to this point. I hope you can see that exercising hard and cutting calories is the problem rather than the solution. It is not a solution to a better body or high blood pressure, insulin resistance, diabetes, cancer, heart disease, etc. Hopefully I have done a good enough job in the preceding chapters to make that point obvious. We have covered the pathophysiology of a modern diet and exercise program, and will be shortly covering ways to work up the problem using modern med-icine, laboratory studies, etc. Now it is time for the resolution. The solution is what I call **RecoverMe**.

Let me start by introducing a new health philosophy or idea that I came up with a few years ago to help people improve their quality of life. It is called **RecoverMe**. **RecoverMe** is a way of life—an attitude, a way of thinking. It conceptualizes possibly the last-ditch effort or possibility for helping people obtain health. What we have been doing and are currently doing is not working. Look around you. Modern medicine, even with all its amazing advancements and technology, including the attempt for universal medical records, Star Wars type surgical procedures, and devices like those of Star Trek's Dr. McCoy to improve diagnosis still have done nothing to help you get that ultimate physique, lose your weight, prevent disease, and improve your quality of life. I mean really improve it. It could certainly be argued that modern medicine does improve quality of life retrospectively. For example, if you lose a limb in a combat situation, modern medicine and technology can provide you with a prosthetic limb, thereby improving your quality of life. Modern medicine can improve your vision if you have cataracts, improve your hearing if you have issues with sound, it can keep you alive after you suffer a massive heart attack—the list goes on.

For mental health conditions such as depression, antidepressants are prescribed—and there is plenty of evidence these don't work. If you are fatigued all the time, legal speed such as Adderall is prescribed. When you can't sleep, sleep aids are prescribed. If you're anxious, antianxiety medications are prescribed. But these meds are bandages and do nothing for your concerns. You still don't feel well—especially when the drugs wear off. A number of these issues present themselves while you are trying to get healthy and are following a rigorous diet and exercise program. Everything you are doing or have done today, if you were lucky helped for a short while, and if you are like the majority of people, did nothing for you.

I mentioned before one of my favorite things to tell my patients: "I can't control your stressors, but I can help your body deal with them better." That is the *RecoverMe* philosophy: help the body recover not only from the diet and exercise program, but from all the stressors on the body—toxins, infections, bad relationships, poor diets, chemicals in your makeup—the list goes on.

Shift work is a great example: Ideally, no one should do shift work, as it really screws up the most important circadian flow of the body. Quitting your job would do nothing but add to the stress, as bills would start to pile up, and dang it, those kids of yours do like to eat! But the *RecoverMe* way of life and ideas will better suit your body to handle that shift work. You can continue your shift work schedule, stay healthy and lean, feel good, and have a good quality of life *IF* you can recover from the shift work schedule.

That leads us into how people piecemeal recovery. Most, if not all, people intuitively know they need to recover and so they pick a few different ways to do it. The following items are the ways most people find recovery:

- Anabolic Steroids
- Pre- and Post-workout Meals
- Nutritional Supplementation
- Diet
- Sleep
- Balance
- Prayer, meditation, spirituality, etc.

These all work, but the correct combination of them is essential for long-term *RecoverMe*. That is an individualized process. Ideally,

I would visit with each one of you reading this book and help you figure out the best path for you to take. From the medical testing, to the personalized eating and exercise plan, right down to the correct supplements to take. As that is obviously not possible, I am listing a lot of information in the next few chapters. Not everything is for everybody. Consider this a reference guide for you and your health care provider to figure out what you need to optimize your health and recover from the effort and work you are putting toward health and that coveted body that got you needing this book in the first place.

We will start by covering the medical evaluation in working up a Fat to Fit problem, and then provide a way to fix it in the following chapters.

A couple of things I feel are important to mention before getting into the next section. The medical evaluation has a lot of testing mentioned. A lot of testing. To be perfectly honest, I can diagnose your overexercising and undereating problem without one drop of blood, one stool sample, or any other testing for that matter. Labs have become more of a commodity and a need based on the advice of Dr. Google. I admit they are fun to do, but in reality, a good doctor should be able to listen to your problems and figure them out, right down to the imbalance of specific hormones. I included this chapter, so you would have a reference point for labs if you do have them done.

In the *RecoverMe* exercise, diet, and supplement section I have made very specific recommendations for a very broad audience. In other words, what I have listed and suggested has worked for a lot of people, but you may need to find what works for you. For example, the eating plan is really good for recovery. But it may not be the one you need for life. The supplement suggestions—something very general like magnesium—may make some people feel great, and others feel terrible. You must try things out and find what works best for you. If you were sitting in my office, I would help you do that. When

I write a book for a larger population, I must lay out several things and trust you to find the combination that works best for you!

# CHAPTER 8
## The Medical Evaluation

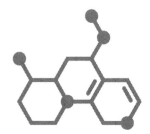

This chapter is not for the lawyers out there. I am not telling you this to cover my backside; I am telling you this because occasionally, there is a concern that needs to be addressed. When you feel as bad as you do after you have been exercising and limited your eating, just like you have been told to do, you need, and your doctor needs, to make sure nothing ominous is going on. It is important. I have caught some serious issues in the workups of people who came to me just feeling awful. I won't go into detail, but suffice it to say, please get yourself checked out when you feel yucky or are gaining weight, even though you are doing everything "right," etc. Thank goodness, it's usually just ramifications of the "healthy" diet and exercise program. Once anything ominous has been ruled out, the next step is to get into more detail about what state your body is currently in so you can fix it. I will break this down for you in slices so you have an idea how to approach it. ***I will not get into detailed explanations of each test.*** That is for your doctor to discuss with you. Different labs have different reference ranges as well. Another reason you need your doctor's involvement. I will give you the basics, with some basic instruction on interpretation, as well as mention a few things I have seen in the past in multiple workups of modern day survivors of overexercising and undereating.

Quick caveat if I may: The following medical workup I will briefly cover may be a bit difficult to grasp. It is a familiarity thing, not reliant at all on how smart you are. It takes years to know what labs to order when someone presents at a doctor's office for evaluation. It takes even longer to know how to interpret those labs. Far too often, I visit with people whose medical provider treated the lab value, but not the patient. Now, I must try to fix him or her, especially in the realms of hormone replacement therapy. That being said—the labs help confirm what I am already thinking. They never make my diagnosis for me and they certainly do not always dictate treatment or intervention.

Testing is fun, as it is neat to see yourself from a different angle or view point. It also is of great benefit if you are stuck. Medical testing, especially labs, should only be done to confirm what your doctor is already thinking—not to make the diagnosis for him or her (broken record, I know). Shotgun approaches are never a good idea with any sort of medical testing, so be sure to check out the doctor's style by talking with previous patrons if you plan to find someone who knows the ins and outs of these tests.

If I were to summarize everything physiologically that I have listed so far in the book as problematic, and the metabolic consequences of most popular diet and exercise programs, here is what the list would look like:

1. **HPA Axis Adversity**
2. **Hormonal Havoc**

3. **Bowel Bollix**
4. **Oxidative Stress**
5. **Toxin Trouble**

As I have already explained why all this occurs, I will use this section to briefly describe medical testing that can be done, and the findings that may/can occur when looking at things in more detail.

Recovering from this condition caused by the diet and exercise program takes time. If I were to throw the proverbial kitchen sink at you to fix you, it would fail. One step at a time is the best and only way to fix this problem. That is why it takes some time, something I cannot reiterate enough in our "I want it **NOW**" society. Enough preaching: let's dive right into some medical testing that can be done to help you see what your get-in-shape program has done to you and give you some insight on how to recover!

I am about to mention a few tests that are of great benefit, as the stage of anarchy your body is in will dictate treatment. For example: the diurnal salivary cortisol test I discuss in the HPA Axis Adversity will show just how far into trouble you are or how your body is responding to the stress you are putting on it. There are different stages of HPA Axis dysfunction, and the treatment is a little different for each stage.

Medical evaluations cost money. Most of the tests described below are not covered or reimbursed by insurance. Just an FYI. If finances are an issue or concern, read this section for information only, and incorporate the ***RecoverMe*** eating plan, exercise program, and suggested supplements as described below, and you will be fine. The testing just allows us to dial in specifics *with greater speed*. I was treating this disorder long before a lot of these tests were available, so I will tell you how to get better with or without the tests! I tell people all the time *"Your wallet is a part of your health. You came to me to get healthy. If I damage your wallet, I am not helping your health at all!"*

Another way to put that is, if you cannot afford the following labs I mention, or there is no doctor in your area who does this kind of testing, you will be OK. The real fix to the damage created modern diet and exercise programs is in the **RecoverMe** section of the book. Labs or not, the use of drugs and/or medication to get better or not—the real fix is what you do every day. That being said, it's also dependent on what you don't do every day—like exercise too much and eat too little!

## Basic Lab Panels Interpreted with Different Glasses

In any workup and review of the symptoms associated and discussed here with your current condition following a trendy exercise and diet plan, most medical providers likely will have some basic tests run, including a Complete Blood Count (CBC) and a Chemistry Panel.

The CBC reveals three things of importance to us in this situation. First, it shows your white cell count and the types/numbers of white cells present. The number of different white blood cells can be an indication to look for inflammatory states, such as those seen with food allergies and other issues that accompany the high-stress load. Looking at eosinophils, monocytes, and basophiles and their absolute count could also give an indication to look further. Second, a red cell count and indices that basically show the size, shape, color, and consistency of the red blood cells. This allows us to diagnose anemia, which is very common in this setting. Third, it shows the hemoglobin and hematocrit, which are basically the amount and percent of the iron-containing, oxygen-carrying portions of the red blood cells. These are important to look at, as they can be low if you're under-recovered and undernourished, or they could be too high if you are using AAS.

A chemistry panel will show kidney and liver function, electrolytes, blood sugar and a few other indicators that point physicians elsewhere if abnormal. Kidney function and liver function can be compromised with a Fat to Fit program, so following these numbers during your recovery is important. Electrolytes can also be off, thanks to the stress and malnourishment involved, so checking those and making sure they are optimal is a must.

It is a good idea for your doctor to run a red blood cell magnesium (RBC Mg+) to make sure this absolutely essential mineral is in your body in the amounts it should be. Magnesium is lacking in our diets and heavy exercisers burn through it like crazy. Checking serum (standard) magnesium is useless, as magnesium is an intra-cellular mineral. Levels should be at least 6.0–6.4 mg/dl for optimal recovery from an overzealous diet and exercise program.

## HPA Axis Adversity

Let's pretend you are sitting in a quiet room reading this book. Suddenly, a saber tooth tiger comes flying through the window next to the chair you're sitting in. You immediately jump up to either start swinging or run like crazy. Your heart is racing, your breath is shallow and quick, your muscles are tense, your blood pressure is up to make sure your brain has enough blood to think, you're jittery and really on edge. Do you fight, or run away? This is the classic fight or flight response your body goes through when confronted with danger. The fight or flight response is mediated by adrenalin and other hormones classified as catecholamines as well as the hormone cortisol.

When you are doing a commonly suggested diet and exercise as you have been doing, your body ends up in a constant state of fight or flight. The intense exercise, in combination with the limited calorie diet, as well as the supplement/drug schedule, results in your body fearing the saber tooth tiger in the room—all the time. That is why you feel horrible all the time. This is why you don't sleep very well—who can sleep with a tiger in their room?

The HPA axis stands for hypothalamic-pituitary-adrenal axis. It is a multifaceted system of hormones that all talk to each other and direct all sorts of activity in the body. Some would consider this group of organs and their associated hormones the master controllers of the body. The H is for hypothalamus. It is in the brain and it controls all the autonomic (automatic) functions of the body in response to the environment. This would include such things as your body temperature, energy, etc. Its job in the axis is to release corticotropin-releasing hormone or CRH. The P is for pituitary and its job in the axis is to release adrenocorticotrophic hormone or ACTH. This gland is also in the brain and releases a whole host of hormones including thyroid-stimulating hormone (TSH), growth hormone (GH), and luteinizing hormone (LH). The A is for the adrenal gland. It produces, among other things, cortisol. It is located above the kidneys and it produces a few other hormones, including adrenalin and DHEA. The combination of CRH-ACTH-cortisol release is referred to as the hypothalamic-pituitary-adrenal axis, or HPA axis. These hormones work via positive and negative feedback loops—in other words, they all talk, with the conversation geared toward keeping cortisol under tight rein and control.

When your body is under stress for more than a few minutes, the hypothalamus releases CRH. CRH tells the pituitary gland to release adrenocorticotrophic hormone or ACTH, which then tells the adrenal gland to release cortisol. CRH and ACTH are released in pulses, which cause continuous release of cortisol from the adrenal gland. Stress results in increased levels of cortisol in the body. Cortisol maintains the fight or flight response by causing blood sugar (glucose) to be released into the blood for quick energy. It also directly affects the gut, the immune system, and the reproductive system. Pain is also modulated via the stress response, as a wonderful chemical called beta-endorphin is released.

Under normal conditions, cortisol release is very circadian and pulsed, based on need. It peaks in the morning upon awakening, nadirs in the late afternoon and slowly rises again to spike in the morning the following day. The circadian pattern of cortisol release is controlled by the suprachiasmatic nucleus of the hypothalamus. Not that you needed to know that, I just like saying it. Of important note—your body clock is located here.

Modern day diet and exercise programs are extremely stress-ful on the body. It causes an overall, if not constant, increase in the release of cortisol. This causes the HPA axis to malfunction and the negative feedback loops no longer have control. Rather than healthy, good for you, pulses of cortisol throughout the day, it becomes chronically elevated.

This causes brain issues, including altering thought processes, thinking, and planning (foggy brain), emotional issues (quick to anger, cry at the slightest thing), etc. All because the brain is trying to regulate or decrease cortisol.

The thyroid becomes negatively affected with constant HPA activation and starts decreasing the release of its hormones. When constantly activated, the HPA axis tempers the immune system, allowing one to become more prone to illness. Inflammation increases in the body because of constant HPA stimulation, as do allergic reac-tions (suddenly, your favorite food causes you belly pain?). The gut starts misbehaving and you develop IBS or irritable bowel syndrome with either constipation or diarrhea—or both (intermittently) (more below in the subsection entitled Bowel Bollix). You lose the ability to handle physical activity, mental loads, and emotional situations. In other words, you fall apart. Interestingly—the same things happen to people with post traumatic stress disorder (PTSD) and chronic fatigue syndrome.

One more quick, nevertheless, frustrating note on high cortisol levels: It causes insulin resistance! Wonder why your weight came back on so quickly following your incredible efforts to get a better body? That is one of the big reasons.

This brings us to how we test the HPA axis. A simple blood panel will not suffice, as your cortisol levels are, as you now understand, greatly influenced by your environment. Many practioners have used a fasting 0800 cortisol level (blood test) to see if it was elevated, but there is a problem with that. Let us say while driving to your doctor's office for the blood test someone cuts you off by running a red light. The result is very elevated levels of cortisol—false reading. Or, even more common, a nurse comes at you with a needle to draw your blood! Being stabbed is stressful to most of us. Elevated cortisol results in a false reading.

We can do something called an ACTH stimulation test to check cortisol levels. You show up at your doctor's office or the hospital lab and they draw your blood. Then they inject you in the shoulder with some ACTH. Then they redraw your blood at 30 or 60 minutes and check your cortisol levels. It is expensive and not used often unless we are looking for something called Addison's disease or true adrenal failure.

The most practical way to test the HPA axis is something called a diurnal salivary cortisol test. This test uses saliva to test two primary hormones in the dysfunction: DHEA and cortisol. It helps us see the pattern of cortisol release over the course of a 24-hour period. Hormones in the saliva are unbound and, therefore, can provide a very accurate assessment of what is going on.

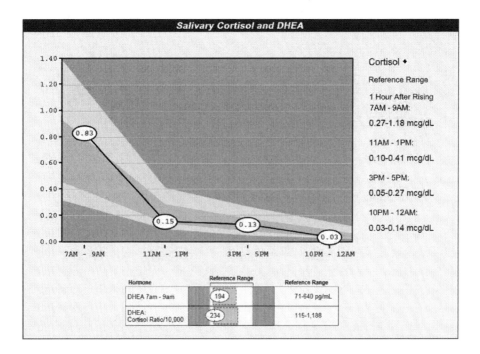

Genova Diagnostic

Without going into detail, this test tells us the current state of your HPA Axis. Cortisol may be high or low. DHEA may be high or low. The ratio of DHEA to Cortisol may be off. I have provided a chart that summarizes highs and lows and then provides some possible interventions to help you—based on the test results. Obviously, to get this information and in turn benefit from the suggested interventions, you will need the test!

Under the **RecoverMe** section of the book, I get into greater detail on most of these.

| *Low Cortisol* | *Suggestions:* | |
|---|---|---|
| | Lifestyle | Quit the Fat to Fit Program! |
| | Nutritional: | Increase your calories |
| | Supplements: | Vitamin C and B-complex a few times a day |
| | Herbal | American ginseng<br>Sarsaparilla<br>Others |
| | Medication | Hormone support and consider glandulars |

| *High Cortisol* | *Suggestions:* | |
|---|---|---|
| | Lifestyle | Quit the Fat to Fit Program!<br>Meditation/prayer<br>Sit in a sauna<br>Fix your gut |
| | Nutritional: | Good balanced diet |
| | Supplements: | Vitamin C and B-complex twice a day<br>Phosphatidylserine at night<br>L-Theanine as needed |
| | Herbal | Passionflower<br>Relora three times a day |
| | Medication | Support other hormones affected by the high cortisol |

| *Low DHEA* | *Suggestions:* | |
|---|---|---|
| *(similar treatment as HIGH cortisol)* | Lifestyle | Quit the Fat to Fit Program!<br>Meditation/prayer<br>Sit in a sauna<br>Fix your gut |
| | Nutritional: | Good balanced diet |
| | Supplements: | Vitamin C and B-complex twice a day<br>Phosphatidylserine at night<br>L-Theanine as needed |
| | Herbal | Passionflower<br>Relora three times a day |
| | Medication | Support other hormones affected by the high cortisol |

| | High DHEA | Suggestions: |
| --- | --- | --- |
| (similar treatment as LOW cortisol) | Lifestyle | Quit the Fat to Fit Program! |
| | Nutritional Supplements: | Increase your calories Vitamin C and B-complex a few times a day |
| | Herbal | American ginseng Sarsaparilla Others |
| | Medication | Hormone support and consider glandulars |

## Hormonal Havoc

As you have been reading, the hormones go into total disarray with the suggested diet and exercise programs the "experts" profess. They are a mess. You know they are a mess. Your friends, if you still have any, know they are a mess. Your family (hopefully you still have one) is is also quite aware that your hormones are jacked! Unfortunately—labs do not always agree.

That is why it is essential to understand the big picture. You must understand the overriding effects of powerful lifestyle hormones including cortisol, as discussed above, leptin, insulin, glucagon, adiponectin, and the brain hormones. These lifestyle related/affected hormones override all the other hormones, such as your thyroid and sex hormones. When you can grasp the fact that the lifestyle hormones are off, it makes sense that the thyroid and sex hormones are off. The combination is why you feel lousy. It is intuitive, as I have already mentioned: evolutionarily, if there is no food or you are constantly under duress and stressed out to the max, nothing that could possibly bring another life into the picture works (your hormones crash, sex drive, and sexual function disappear, so you don't/can't have kids). End of story.

I wrote out several different ways to cover this—all of them were a bit too wordy, so I narrowed it down to a simple list or panel to have your doctor check, and what to look for. Having read the above, you know why I order these tests, so let us review them with a little more detail.

Yet another caveat (seems to be a lot of those when you deal with human beings!), there are patterns that evolve when looking at these tests. That is hard to describe in text or verbally, for that matter. Try to explain the exact geometry of a spider's web. Or the fractal formed by freezing water. You cannot. Looking at labs in this setting, the same things happen. Over the years, I started to see patterns evolve that showed me the direction to go. Can I explain that to you or another doctor for that matter? Yes, I can. But it is difficult as I am not that verbally fluent. I can give you some basics and suggest some things you can try, with the help of your medical provider.

This also means that a lot of the labs may fall into the "WNL" or Within Normal Limits realm. Hormone normal ranges are wide, depending on when the lab was taken (time of day, time of month, etc.) That is why patterns are so important. One lab test that is WNL, but on the high side of its range, compared to a lab test WNL, on the low side of its range, is a pattern that may be indicative of an issue. One cannot rely just on lab tests that fall outside WNL.

## Hormones 101

Hormones are chemical messengers carried by blood to non-adjacent target cells. They regulate growth and development and they control homeostasis, which is the regulation of internal environment all by parameters maintained within relatively narrow limits. They control reproductive systems and processes, such as ovulation, menstruation, and maintenance of pregnancy. They affect behavior via modification, modulation, and initiation of specific patterns. In short: Hormones are messengers. They all talk.

Western medicine, I believe, views them inappropriately, as they put them in boxes just as they do every other system in the body. Let me give you an example: as hormones are messengers, let's use the analogy of a mailperson again. Let's say you live in New York, and I live in Idaho. I write you a letter telling you the dangers of the diet and exercise program you are doing. I give it to the messenger (the mailperson). He passes it to the messenger in Wyoming, who shares it with the gal in Iowa, who then gives it to the guy in Illinois, who happens to be a daytime drinker. He loses my letter. Western medicine would come to you and ask why you did not get the letter. The focus is on the beginning and the end—nothing between—hence, a lot of hormonal issues are missed. I think it's best to understand the messengers themselves, as well as how they interact with others. You know—kindergarten social instruction. Let me give you a visual analogy:

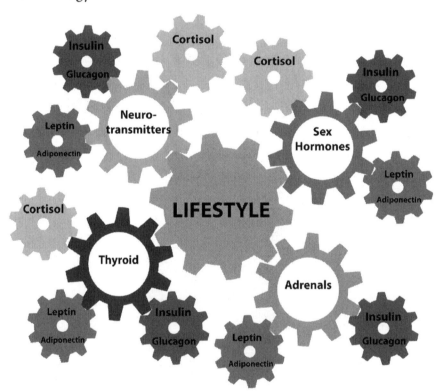

When one hormone moves with this cog-wheel analogy, it changes the others or makes them move. One hormone cannot be muddled with, changed, added to, or taken away without affecting another one. For example, if you look up and to the left of the picture you can see the neurotransmitters are influenced by the lifestyle hormones leptin, adiponectin, insulin, glucagon, and cortisol (which also directly affect your adrenals, your sex hormones, and your thyroid function). The change in neurotransmitters, now "moves" or makes changes to your lifestyle, that then also indirectly affects your sex hormones, thyroid, and adrenals.

Modern/popular diet and exercise programs increase cortisol, for example, and affects every other hormone in your body, which then has influence on your lifestyle, that then affects your other hormones. They cannot be separated or looked at as distinct, individually functioning hormones. If your doctor replaces your testosterone (or thyroid, or DHEA, or any hormone for that matter), but does not consider the other hormones being provoked, other issues will start to occur including new symptoms or concerns and/or the sense that the hormone that was replaced no longer works.

As grasping an understanding of this is so very important, let me use another analogy:

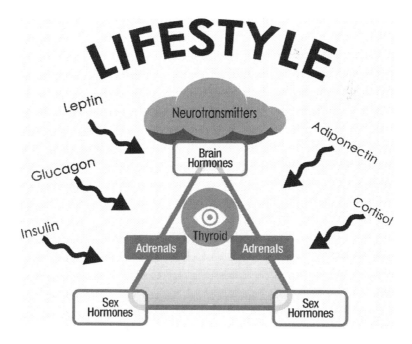

Let us say your hormones are a pyramid. There is a cloud above the pyramid—that represents your brain neurotransmitters/hormones. When they are in a storm, everything below gets rained on and does not work very well. The top of the pyramid is hypothalamus and pituitary. They send hormonal messages to everyone below, controlling a lot of functions and activities, but also responding to information from the hormones below (feedback loop). The eye of the pyramid is your thyroid—involved in everything metabolically that your body does. Two structural components on the pyramid are your adrenal glands, and at the base of the pyramid are your sex hormones.

A large stone ball rolls up and down the four-sided pyramid in response to the environment. When one hormone gets off, the ball gets stuck and the other hormones don't respond/work as well.

The real kicker is the fact that the hormone pyramid sits in your lifestyle hormones. Leptin, adiponectin, insulin, glucagon, and cortisol—all the hormones that respond to and then help control your lifestyle environment override the hormone pyramid. When these lifestyle hormones go wacky because of your lifestyle (in our case, the overexercising and undereating), the whole pyramid is off. The labs might look normal on paper when tested, but because they are sitting in the screwed-up lifestyle hormones, they don't work! Keep this in mind, as I describe the following hormone tests and interventions—it will make more sense.

**Remember—these are all being explained in the setting of someone trying really hard to improve their physique so I have listed them using the hormonal pyramid as my guide. There are multiple causes for a few of the hormonal peculiarities I will explain, but to emphasize:** *I am only covering the reasons appli-cable to the situation we are discussing now.* **For example, DHEA-s may be low if someone is taking antiepileptic drugs. I am not cov-ering seizure disorders in this book or several of the reasons a lab may be off. That is your doctor's job.**

## Basic Hormonal Panel for Females and Males

I am listing the male and female hormone panels together. For a workup following (or during) a common diet and exercise program, they are essentially the same. Of course, there are several other tests I could do in a female vs. a male, but back to the point of the book.

Females are a bit more complicated than males—nothing personal, as a matter of fact—it's a compliment! The first thing you must do, when evaluating a woman's hormones, is know where she is in her menstrual cycle. If she is menopausal, do not worry. You can draw labs anytime of the month. If she should be menstruating and is not, tough luck—hormone panels will be harder to read. If she is still cycling, you want to know *exactly* where she is in her cycle before you test. If she does know, there are two times I like best: Day 1–3 of her cycle (days 1–3 of actual bleeding) or days 19–25 of her cycle (luteal phase). Some might benefit from measuring at ovulatory time or mid-cycle. These times are obvious to women. At least the prior one is. Some women cannot tell when they ovulate, while others can by pain, temperature change, vaginal discharge changes, etc. When testing is done, you must control for the variability of the monthly cycle. One should also control for the time of day and food. That goes for men, too. Labs should be done first thing in the morning (no exercise before), fasting, at a known time of month for women.

## Psych Hormones

Following (or during) a "going for the gusto" diet and exercise program, most of your brain hormones are off. In many instances, the precursor nutrients to neurotransmitters are lacking due to the eating plan. High cortisol from the stress of the program destroys nerve connections and causes neuronal death. Changes in peripheral hormones change the brain hormones—DHEA for example, high or low, causes memory issues. There are tests we can do to look at neurotransmitters. I, for one, do not really use or rely on testing them—I know they are off, as it is obvious when someone presents to my clinic. If you want them tested, it can be done, but it really does not change how we fix them (most of the time) as the fix involves optimizing the lifestyle and controlling the "other" hormones.

## Brain Hormones

### Follicle-Stimulating Hormone (FSH) and Luteinizing Hormone (LH)

These hormones have different roles in men and women. In women, FSH stimulates the ovary to produce hormones—estradiol during the follicular phase and progesterone during the luteal phase of each menstrual cycle. In men, FSH stimulates Sertoli cells in the testicles to make sperm. LH in women stimulates the ovary to make steroid hormones as well, and surges mid-cycle to trigger ovulation. LH in men stimulates Leydig cells to produce testosterone.

#### *FSH and LH are low*

In a strenuous physique-altering program, if these brain hormones are low it is very likely because he or she has been using drugs such as anabolic androgenic steroids (AAS) or the variety of prohormones out there. Excessive hormones based on testosterone decrease these brain hormones to a mere nothing.

They are also low in the setting of excessive exercise and high levels of cortisol found in someone doing a modern diet and exercise program. Low levels of progesterone can also lower these brain hormones.

#### *FSH and LH are elevated*

Later along the time line from doing a demanding diet and exercise program, these labs can become elevated. If drugs were used for the program, the drugs could have knocked out the body's ability to make its own hormones—it is rare, but I have seen it (especially in men on AAS). Extremely high levels of insulin from the rebound pig-out sessions that follow certain diet and exercise programs can increase LH. A man or woman taking the fertility drug Clomid—clomiphene—can also elevate these hormones. Clomiphene is used by men and women as PCT—post-cycle therapy—following the use of AAS.

## Prolactin

Prolactin is a pituitary hormone named for the fact that it causes milk let down in mammals. It has a few other functions in the body, including metabolic, behavior, immune function, and fluid regulation. It is also produced in several other places in the body, but that is beyond the scope of this book.

*Prolactin is low*

A low level can indicate hyperthyroidism. This can be an autoimmune condition or from taking too much thyroid medication. Bulimia in someone who has chosen another extreme to get the body they want also can show low prolactin levels.

*Prolactin is high*

High levels occur after someone stops their thyroid medication they used to try to get in better shape and has slipped into hypothyroidism. Low blood sugars from insulin use or just low calories can do it as well.

## Thyroid-Stimulating Hormone (TSH)

Thyroid-stimulating hormone tells the thyroid to produce hormones. It is a "growth hormone" for the thyroid, if you will. It, like most brain hormones, works on a feedback loop. It is the opposite of what one would think—If TSH is low, your thyroid is producing too much or you are taking too much hormone. If TSH is high, your brain is asking your thyroid to produce more hormone or your doctor needs to prescribe more thyroid hormone.

### TSH is low

In a modern diet and exercise program this is rare, unless prescription drugs such as Cytomel, Synthroid, or Levothyroxine (or any of the thyroid medications) are being utilized and overdone.

### TSH is high

This is much more common. If the level is greater than 2 IU/mL, in my opinion, it is too high (normal by my lab is 0.3–3.0 IU/mL). This can be elevated due to stress (as discussed above), rebound effects from inappropriate thyroid medication use that was stopped abruptly, or the start of an auto-immune process called autoimmune thyroiditis or Hashimoto's disease, due to a ruined gut (we will talk about this later).

## Thyroid Hormones

The thyroid produces T4 (less active hormone) and T3, the more active hormone. All of the T4 is converted to T3 in the body. T4 is needed for the brain, as it can cross the blood brain barrier, T3 cannot. T3 is the fuel for the mitochondria—the "powerhouses" of the cells in the body. So, in the presence of any energy issue, this hormone needs to be looked at closely.

### Triiodothyronine (Free T3) is low

This takes some defining of the word "low" (not quite unlike President Clinton to define the word "is"). In the overexercising, undereating setting, if you were paying attention as you read above, high cortisol levels (high stress) negatively affect T3. Therefore, in this setting, a "normal" range Free T3 is not normal if it is less than 3.5 (normal range by my lab is 2.4–4.2 pg/mL). Anything below 3.5 pg/mL needs to be treated, either by lowering cortisol, changing leptin kinetics, or adding medication in the short term. Recall what I said above: When T3 is low, nutrient absorption is decreased by up to 50%, so intervention is needed sooner rather than later when this lab comes up abnormal.

For some reason, I see a lot of autoimmune thyroiditis or Hashimoto's Disease in chronic dieters (likely due to gut issues or toxins)—this can also cause low thyroid numbers even in the face of a normal TSH.

**Triiodothyronine (Free T3) is high**

If this is the case, and in the realms we have been discussing, three scenarios are possible: You are a teenager, as teenagers have high T3 levels; you are still taking your Cytomel or some other thyroid replacement; or you have an overactive thyroid—a condition called Graves' disease.

**Thyroxine (T4) is low**

T4 can be low coming off thyroid drugs, or you are not taking enough if you are on prescription drugs. It can also be low in the setting of autoimmune disease—something called autoimmune thyroiditis or Hashimoto's Disease (see above).

## Thyroid Peroxidase Antibody (TPO)

TPO tests for autoantibodies against your thyroid. We use it in medicine as one of many tests to distinguish thyroid dysfunction. When it is elevated, it means your immune system has started to recognize your thyroid as a bad guy and attacks it. As I have mentioned throughout the book, an overexercising, undereating program causes havoc galore and causes all sorts of things to go haywire—this is one I see often. Gluten is often implicated in the presence of a "leaky gut" (see below) as the trigger that turns the immune system on your thyroid. This is an important test, as optimal thyroid function is essential for recovery from a modern diet and exercise program.

## ReverseT3

rT3 is a metabolite of T4 (thyroxine). Under healthy circumstances, T4 has iodine removed and becomes T3—the active hormone. In high-stress, high-cortisol situations, with altered leptin kinetics, T4 can be converted to rT3. Think of rT3 as the broken version of T3. If rT3 is high normal or high, greater than 15 ng/dl, you have a thyroid problem. This test is important, as following a Fat to Fit program, TSH and T4 levels are poor indicators of actual thyroid function at the level of the cell. A low Free T3 with a high to normal rT3, a low or high T4, and a normal TSH is a very classic picture of the thyroid dysfunction following a valiant attempt to change your body.

There are some arguments about using or determining the ratio of Free T3 to rT3. There are 20 different interpretations of this ratio and, since the units used need to be the same (ng/dL or pmol/L or pg/mL, etc.), it can become confusing. That is why I described what I did above: if you have a low Free T3, <3.5 pg/mL, and an rT3 greater than 15 ng/dL, there is an issue.

## Progesterone

Progesterone is a very important hormone. In medical schools, soon-to-be doctors are taught that progesterone is the hormone of pregnancy (PRO-Gestation = PROgesterone) and causes the uterine lining to sluff off for menstruation if there is no fertilized egg present. That's it.

As nothing is ever that simple, progesterone's roles are manifold. It is the precursor to several other hormones, it works as an antianxiety drug in anxious women (current diet and exercise recommendation survivors), and is one of the best sleep aids I have ever prescribed!

Time of the month is essential for this test, so if the woman is not menstruating, due to age or the effects of the diet and exercise program she is doing, it will be harder to interpret. This is one test on the list I will occasionally run for men, but since I do not do it frequently, I will focus on the girls.

**Progesterone is low**

Chronic stress lowers this one. Strenuous exercise and limited eating, oral contraceptives and a few antibiotics all can lower progesterone. As a woman rapidly gains weight following her attempts to lose it, her estrogen may take off, leaving progesterone in the dust. If this is the case, she becomes estrogen dominant, which is demonstrated by excessive and painful bleeding, tender breasts, and emotionally daft. Cortisol also competes for progesterone receptors, so high stress most certainly affects this hormone.

**Progesterone is high**

This may be seen early on in a crazy diet an exercise program with extreme adrenal hyperactivity, as your body tries to keep up with your self-induced stress. Things that inhibit progesterone metabolism may also be playing a role, such as cigarette smoke, or certain antacids (cimetidine).

## Sex Hormone Binding Globulin (SHBG)

SHBG is a protein made by the liver that, as the name implies, binds hormones, specifically testosterone and estrogen. A few conditions, drugs, toxins, etc. all change the way this guy works, so it is essential it be checked in a hormonal work up.

**SHBG low**

Thyroid depression from the activities of a forceful exercise and extreme dieting lowers this, as do high insulin levels. The nightly bender of vodka after you crash and burn from your program also lowers it. Taking testosterone or other AAS can lower it as well. The weight gain from high insulin (chicken or the egg?), from the eating that occurs after you throw in the towel on your body efforts—even if it is within reason—can lower SHBG and, therefore, free up more testosterone. In the case of women, this tends to show up as midlife acne and midline hair (chin, nipples, bellybutton to pubic bone, inner thighs), that appear out of nowhere, and just adds to their frustration.

**SHBG high**

Thyroid medication taken by body worshipers can raise this, as can the significant initial weight loss they experienced with the dangerous diet and exercise program. Extremes of caffeine—very common—can raise this, as can a few of the drugs occasionally used by those attempting to get the perfect body, including clomiphene and tamoxifen.

## Dehydroepiandrosterone Sulfate (DHEA-s)

DHEA-s is a vitally important hormone in both men and women. It is produced by the adrenal glands, gonads, and the brain. It has many roles in the body, including being a precursor hormone to a number of other hormones.

**DHEA is low**

Chronic stress of a modern diet and exercise program lowers this, as does chronic inflammation.

**DHEA is high**

This is seen in insulin resistance as well as acute stress as with severe caloric restriction. Taking DHEA supplements can increase it as can the use of clomiphene.

## Total and Free Testosterone

Testosterone is a key player in life. It gets a lot (if not all) of the credit and/or blame for everything sexual; however, that is not fair to the hormone. Yes—it is involved with sex drive and sexual function, but so is every other hormone in your body. Your mood, how you feel about yourself or your mate, etc. all play a role in you wanting (or not wanting) sex. The biggest sex organ in your body is between your ears. Testosterone is a very complex hormone with so many actions I cannot list them all here. In short: testosterone, in balance with the other hormones, is essential to recover from an overdone diet and exercise program. Total testosterone should be reviewed in women and free or bioavailable testosterone should be reviewed in men (along with total). There are more and more labs and physicians changing to "age dependent lab ranges" which I think will add a lot of value and more understanding to the test and its implications. As this is not universally accepted as of yet, I will focus on just "high" or "low" and let you and your doctor determine that within the clinical presentation.

**Testosterone is low**

It may be low in this setting, due to the use of hormones or prohormones if done prior to the test. Taking hormones from the outside lower your own production (or turn it off). A high inflammatory state lowers it, as does high conversion to estrogen, or what we call high aromatase activity. Aromatase activity is increased in excessive alcohol use and increasing belly fat, as it has a high amount of aromatase activity. A few specific medications can lower it, including a diuretic often used for physique shows called spironolactone. Marijuana users may also find themselves with low testosterone levels. High cortisol levels and a high degree of stress also lowers it.

**Testosterone is high**

In this particular setting, taking testosterone at the time of the test would obviously make this number high. There are a few other conditions that do it, but that is beyond the scope of this book. Testosterone, like most things in life, is on a bell-shaped curve. When you have too much testosterone, your symptoms are very similar to those appearing when you do not have enough.

## Estradiol (E2)

Estradiol is one of three estrogens in your body. In men and women, high levels occur due to over conversion of testosterone (androgens) to estrogen in belly fat. It is obviously involved in what makes a woman a woman, and it is important in both men and women for sexual health, vascular health, bone health, and brain health.

**Estradiol is low**

Early on, during or soon after a rigorous diet and exercise pro-gram, E2 is low. This is due to low body weight, strenuous exercise, chronic stress on the body, chronic inflammation from the program, etc. This will cause all sorts of emotional issues, such as low libido, poor sexual function (poor lubrication and a difficult time with orgasm), anovulation (so no menstrual cycle), etc. Also, if you have had a hysterectomy or even a tubal ligation for birth control, your estrogen can be low especially in this setting.

In men, this is found when they are taking aromatase inhibitors like Arimidex. It also can cause the same symptoms discussed above that occur in women (except the menstrual changes) and is really concerning, as E2 protects the cardiac blood vessels from damage. Too low a level of E2 in a man, and he is a heart attack waiting to happen.

**Estradiol is high**

Changes in conversion and clearance via the liver and intestinal beta-glucuronidase activity increase estrogen in both men and women following a Fat to Fit program. High estrogen also occurs in the setting of a dysfunctional thyroid, high inflammatory states (cytokines increase conversion of E1 to E2), and or AAS use in both men and women.

## Insulin Growth Factor-1 (IGF-1)

IGF-1 is a polypeptide hormone released primarily by the liver in response to the brain's production of growth hormone. Growth hormone is released in spurts. Testing it is a moving target, as one never knows when it is spurting. Therefore, we look indirectly at growth hormone via the steadier state released hormone IGF-1. IGF-1 is an anabolic hormone like insulin.

**IGF-1 is low**

IGF-1 tends to be decreased, like all anabolic hormones, in the presence of modern day diet and exercise suggestions due to high-stress states, inflammatory cytokines, lack of sleep, etc. I have found that, when it is low in individuals, increasing the production of growth hormone via optimal diet and exercise amounts, and possibly even a stimulating peptide, makes a big difference in recovery.

### IGF-1 is high

This occurs when human growth hormone (hGH) or a hGH stimulant is being used. It is also elevated in pregnancy or with a pituitary tumor.

## Adiponectin

Adiponectin is adipokine, meaning it is a hormone released from fat cells, particularly abdominal/visceral fat. It is a powerful marker of disease, particularly diabetes and insulin resistance and cardiovascular disease. One would think that, as it is released by fat, the more fat you have, the more you would release. This is not true in the case of adiponectin. The more abdominal fat one has, the lower the adiponectin level tends to be. It is a little hard to understand, as adiponectin levels are also low in lean people. The fact is, low levels, no matter what the cause, tend to be problematic.

There are "normal" levels designated on body composition or body mass index (BMI), but their ranges are wide, as all "normal" hormone levels are.

### Adiponectin is low

Following an overexercising, undereating program, adiponectin tends to be low, likely due to the low body fat levels. Unfortunately, as weight is gained, adiponectin stays low and all sorts of issues follow. Low levels of adiponectin are associated with inflammation, bad cholesterol numbers, insulin resistance and increased risk of diabetes, non-alcoholic fatty liver disease or NAFLD, coronary heart disease, and cancer. It also has a role in helping your body utilize/burn fat—thereby the harder you try, the less adiponectin is made, and the fat burning stops.

I have found that with levels less than 14 mcg/mL, the fat burning stops, insulin resistance is occurring, and people with levels below this struggle to find energy.

A few ways to increase adiponectin include a few pharmaceutical drugs, such as the blood pressure medicine ACE inhibitors. Supplements such as fish oil, conjugated linoleic acid (CLA), grapeseed extract, green tea extract, the amino acid taurine, and resveratrol have also shown some promise in increasing adiponectin. A good, nutritionally and calorically adequate eating plan with appropriate exercise also increase adiponectin.

**Adiponectin is high**

This is a good thing. I have never seen it following a Fat to Fit program, but it should be a goal of yours to get your adiponectin levels as high as you can!

# Insulin

Insulin is one of the five lifestyle hormones. Insulin levels are of great importance in helping make the diagnosis of an overexercising, undereating issue and in following how well someone is doing in recovery. Like other hormones discussed, there is an optimal level of fasting insulin in the body. Some people have naturally higher levels, as they are likely high secretors of insulin. These are ("big" is a generalization here) your "bigger" people: born big and have big bones, big frames, etc., possibly due to in-utero exposure to high insulin levels. When you secrete insulin after a meal is also very important. Early secretors tend to have more insulin issues (insulin resistance, PECOS, etc.) than slow secretors. This can be discovered using a glucose tolerance test with insulin levels. This test has you drink (or eat) a 75-gram glucose load and check your blood sugars and insulin levels at 30 min, 1 hour, and 2 hour marks. It can be very helpful in diagnosing insulin resistance and early insulin secretion following a meal.

An ideal and healthy level is between 6 and 8 mIU/L. In thin or lean, healthy looking people, one can have normal insulin levels, normal fasting blood sugar levels, yet still be insulin resistant—one of the primary reasons your fat came back so quickly after you worked so hard to lose it. This is in part due to your ruined/leaky gut and direct injury to the pancreatic B-cells where insulin is made. This is also why I stress doing several tests and looking at the big picture as your doctor can not make a diagnosis based on the results of one test.

**Insulin is low**

When insulin levels are too low, defined as less than 5 mIU/L, one is hungry, fatigued and, in general—not fun to be around. This is a very common finding in the overexercising, undereating population, especially women! Sorry girls.

**Insulin is high**

When insulin is greater than 11 mIU/L, we are getting into the early insulin resistance range and it is, therefore, harder to burn fat.

# Leptin

Leptin, as I have mentioned a few times above, is a mother hormone. It is one of the five lifestyle hormones, and one that likely tends to take over and override many other hormones and their functions. I will not spend too much time on leptin here as I have covered it already.

Leptin needs to be measured first thing in the morning in a fasting state. Leptin is very circadian and likely peaks at 0200 or so, while sleeping, but I can never get anyone in for a blood draw at that time, so for the first thing in the morning, reading is a good starting point.

Leptin, like adiponectin, has a few reference ranges based on age, sex, body fat, and even maturity rate (called Tanner staging) in kids and early adolescents. As I did with adiponectin, I will narrow it down, as the modern diet and exercise population has several similarities and, ideally, we get everyone to a BMI of between 18 and 25. As with insulin, it should be interpreted in a range for both men and women. Anything outside of this range, and we have issues with all of the other hormones! Leptin should be between 5 and 10 ng/mL for men and 8–15 ng/mL for women.

**Leptin is low**

When leptin levels are low, one experiences constant hunger, mood concerns, and, as we have already discussed, all your other hormones stop functioning properly (thyroid, testosterone, etc.). This is very commonly seen following a forceful diet and exercise program and in conjunction with low insulin levels. It basically means you need to eat more and exercise less so all the other hormones balance out and start working!

**Leptin is high**

When leptin levels are elevated, you become leptin resistant and the same thing occurs—hunger, moods, and complete hormonal disarray. High cortisol levels cause leptin resistance in the brain so understanding cortisol in this setting is optimal.

# SUMMARY

Admittedly, this was a short review of hormones and the hormonal havoc that occurs with a modern-day diet and exercise program. I hope it provides you with enough information to know what to ask a hormone specialist in your area when you go in for a consultation.

Below is a list of the hormones I just reviewed in chart form for quick reference:

| Pyramid Site | Hormone Test | Sample Type/test |
|---|---|---|
| Brain Hormones | LH | Blood |
| | FSH | Blood |
| | TSH | Blood |
| | Prolactin | Blood |
| | IGF-1 | Blood |
| Thyroid hormones | Total T3 and T4 | Blood |
| | Free T3 and T4 | |
| | Reverse T3 | Blood |
| | TPO | Blood |
| Mid-level hormones /Adrenal hormones | DHEA-s | Saliva, Blood |
| | Cortisol | Blood, saliva |
| Bottom of the pyramid hormones | Total and free testosterone | Blood, saliva, urine |
| | Estradiol | Blood, saliva, urine |
| | Progesterone | Blood, saliva, urine |
| | SHBG | Blood |
| Lifestyle hormones | Leptin | Blood |
| | Insulin | Blood |
| | Adiponectin | Blood |

## Bowel Bollix

Not everyone who has done or is currently doing an exercise and diet program has gut *symptoms*. By symptoms I mean bloating, excessive gas, pain, reflux, constipation or diarrhea (sometimes both intermittently), etc. But everyone who has done or is doing a hardcore diet and exercise program has gut *issues*! It is inevitable, as the extremely high cortisol levels, nutritional deficiencies, and occasional supplements and drugs cause gut dysfunction. This is very important, as you need to have a good functioning gut for all the hormones we mentioned above to work.

Gut issues resolve over time when one incorporates the *RecoverMe* program I will discuss soon. But, as I mentioned above, testing allows us to get there more quickly and accurately. I will just briefly review my favorite gut tests, as I think they do just that: get us to a solution more quickly.

## The Poop Test:

Yes—this is a poop test, not a crappy test, but one in which you collect your stool in what looks like a tater-tot bucket from a fast food restaurant. Sounds fun, I know, but is worth the pain, and smell, and occasional vomit in your mouth from the dry-heaves This test allows us to really look at the gut *function*—something your standard gastroenterologist (GI doc) does not do. Don't get me wrong—GI docs are awesome. It is a tough system to deal with. Most of their tests are anatomical—looking at the anatomy of the gut (with cameras in both of your gut tube orifices) not the actual function.

## Digestion/Absorption Indicators

Digestion/absorption indicators are important. With the broken gut lining that can occur from excessive exercise and unhealthy eating we need to make sure you have digestive enzymes and are absorbing your proteins and fats. In other words, we are making sure there is not a lot of protein and fat in your poop.

## Gut Immunology

We look at markers of inflammation and use this test to help distinguish autoimmune disorders such as ulcerative colitis from irritable bowel syndrome (IBS). It also tells us to look for signs of infection, too much ibuprofen use (or any anti-inflammatory drug), and cancer. We also look for signs of food allergies and determine if more testing may be needed.

## Gut bugs

We use this test to look at all the microbiota in the gut. Do you have good or bad bacteria in there? Are there any really bad bugs or yeast causing problems, etc.?

## Metabolic Indicators

These are the prebiotics you may be familiar with. Bug food or probiotic food if you will. To have good bugs, you need good food. A lot of current diet and exercise programs have very little fiber (the source of short chain fatty acids (SCFA) which is what the good bugs like to eat). This is the best way to tell if we need to supplement fiber or increase it in the lifestyle diet.

## Food Sensitivity Testing

With many overzealous eating plans, food sources remain pretty constant and can potentially, in the face of a "leaky gut" caused by the high cortisol and stress on the body, start to cause your immune system to recognize the foods you are eating on a regular basis as bad guys. This can lead to food sensitivities via something called molecular mimicry. The immune system is triggered by a food source (antigen) and develops an army (antibodies) that then goes on the attack in other parts of your body. A great example is gluten causing your immune system to attack your thyroid —autoimmune thyroiditis (found by looking at TPO, as mentioned above).

## Gut Integrity Markers

I am sure you have heard the term "leaky gut." It is also called increased intestinal permeability which means things are getting past your protective gut lining that should not be getting past. All of the above tests indicate a leaky gut, but there are tests that specifically test to see if leaky gut is present. These include a urine test, in which the first urine sample of the morning, after a night of fasting, is collected, then a prefabbed drink with lactulose and mannitol (two sugars that are not absorbed normally by the gut) with another urine test 6 hours later is done and these sugars are looked for. A blood or stool test called Zonulin is newer to the market and also tests for leaky gut. There are a few others as well, but my experience with them is limited.

## Oxidative Stress

Oxidative stress is basically a disparity between the production of free radicals and the ability of the body to respond to or detoxify their harmful effects through nullification by antioxidants.

Oxidation means the removal of electrons from an atom or molecule. These electrons build up over time and can start damaging your system. The best example I can think of is leaving your dad's new shovel out in the rain—the rust that subsequently occurs is oxidative damage. This is a normal by-product of metabolism, but over time, and in stressful conditions, it starts damaging your body. Every organ and system in your body is damaged by oxidative stress. Oxidative stress causes heart disease, as well as skin changes, such as wrinkling and age marks. It causes kidney disease, arthritis, and other joint issues. Eye damage in the form of macular degeneration and cataracts is a form of oxidative stress. Auto-immune diseases, lung diseases, and brain issues/diseases can all have some of their roots traced back to oxidative stress.

A contemporary diet and exercise program is seething with oxidative stress via all the mechanisms mentioned above, from the overexercising and undereating, and a few of the supplements and drugs.

You can assume you are high in oxidative stress following a serious diet and exercise program, or you can test for it using a few markers. I would not suggest you do all the tests listed below but rather, with the help of your doctor, choose the ones that might be most pertinent to you and your situation. For example; if you are a 50-year-old Fat to Fit survivor with a family history of heart disease, you may want to look at oxLDL and MPO. If you are a younger, active 25-year-old, stressed out to the hilt because you cannot get the body you want, you should do the 8OHdG test.

Once again, it is way beyond the scope of this book to describe each one in great detail, as we are focused on the problem and the recovery, but if you are interested in how much oxidative stress you have in your system, the following is a list of tests you can do to help you measure/follow for your recovery:

- oxLDL
    - 0 oxLDL occurs when the LDL cholesterol particles in your body react with free radicals. The more free radicals, the more oxLDL. These particles then begin reacting with surrounding tissues, causing damage, especially in the arteries. This is immediately followed by the accumulation of inflammatory cells, such as macrophages, and makes the area sticky so more and more inflammatory particles start to build up. Eventually, you have vascular disease and issues such as heart disease, dementia, etc. This is a simple blood test your doctor can run for you.
- Urine levels of microalbumin
    - 0 Microalbumin is a protein found in the urine that represents kidney damage from oxidative stress. It can also be found in cases of kidney infections, high fevers, high blood pressure, heart disease, etc. The best way to test for it is a 24-hour urine catch.

- 8-hydroxydeoxyguanosine (8-OHdG)

    o In nuclear and mitochondrial DNA, 8-OHdG is an oxidized nucleoside of DNA. After oxidative damage, when the DNA starts to repair itself, 8-OHdG is excreted in the urine. Studies have shown that urinary 8-OHdG is not only a great biomarker of generalized, cellular oxidative stress, but also a marker/risk factor for cancer, heart disease (atherosclerosis), and diabetes.

- SOD1 and SOD2

    o The SOD1 gene provides instructions for making an enzyme called superoxide dismutase. This enzyme binds to molecules of copper and zinc to break down toxic, charged oxygen molecules called superoxide radicals. These molecules are by-products of normal cell metabolism, but are increased in the presence of high oxidative stress—such as those that ensue an irrational diet and exercise program. When they are not broken down, cellular damage starts to occur. Superoxide dismutase-2 (SOD2) is a mitochondrial enzyme that scavenges oxygen radicals produced by the extensive oxidation-reduction and electron transport reactions occurring in mitochondria.

- Myeloperoxidase (MPO)

    o MPO is a white blood cell-derived inflammatory enzyme that is used in assessing someone's cardiovascular risk. When an artery wall is damaged from a high inflammatory state, MPO is released. MPO is believed to mediate the vascular inflammation that causes plaque build-up in the arteries. So, your diet and exercise program that was to make you a lean mean healthy machine, and the resulting high oxidative stress, puts you at risk for future heart disease. This test will help you and your doctor quantify your risk.

- Gamma-glutamyl transferase (GGT)

    0 GGT is a liver function test that gives doctors an indication of liver disease and/or helps them quantify other disease processes in the body. Elevated levels of GGT are a simple, but accurate measure of oxidative stress in the body.

- Lipopolysaccharides (LPS)

    0 Lipopolysaccharides (LPS), also known as lipoglycans and endotoxins (mentioned above), are large molecules consisting of a lipid and a polysaccharide. It is produced by gram negative bacteria (and is part of the cell wall of these bacteria). Under stressful situations, and as part of the cellular stress response, superoxide is encouraged by LPS and the resulting damage can be significant. LPS has been indicated in insulin resistance in thin, healthy-looking people, like someone doing one of these popular Internet based diet and exercise programs.

- pH of less than 6.8 in urine and saliva (see below)

    0 Salivary and urinary pH is a great and very inexpensive way to measure the condition and function of the body. I spend a few more sentences discussing it below.

## Toxin Trouble

One thing that may be considered good about a Fat to Fit program is the fact that toxins are not usually an obvious issue. Heavy sweating, saunas, and the avoidance of processed foods really help to minimize common, everyday toxins in regular users. I am mentioning it here because, if you and your doctor get stuck in your recovery, it may be something to consider. Now that your body is a wreck from the overexercising and undereating, toxins could potentially be causing chaos.

A 1987 study by the Environmental Protection Agency (EPA) stated that the average American has at least seven hundred (700) toxins in their body. That was 1987. Currently (as of 2016), there are more than 85,000 chemicals in our everyday products in the US and, other than medications and some pesticides, not very many have been tested for human safety. In 1987, 700 toxins; 30 years later, in 2017, for those of us over that age, how many do we have in us now?

Remember what I said in Chapter 2? Toxins are stored in your fat. After a Fat to Fit program, you have shrunk your fat cells, thus releasing several of these toxins into your body. Could that be why you feel so lousy following a program that was supposed to make you feel good? It is certainly a possibility and, hence, why I am mentioning it.

Toxins build up in your system due either to exposure or to your body's inability to clear them. Toxins come from drugs (prescription, recreational, over-the-counter, etc.), food additives and preservatives (too many protein shakes?), infections, alcohol, tobacco, air pollution, ionizing radiation, electromagnetic waves (too much time on your cell phone?), etc.

Your body's inability to clear them can be due to lung issues, such as asthma, nasal issues like chronic sinusitis, issues with bowel movements (constipation), or your mental/emotional coping skills with stressors, such as a bad relationship, your dislike of your God-given body, or a common diet and exercise program.

Let me give you a few specific examples. Most, if not all, diet and exercise programs encourage drinking water. That is great, but how do most of us (me included, especially when I am in a hurry) drink our water? Out of plastic containers. The stereotypical picture of a bodybuilder carrying his or her gallon milk jug full of water everywhere they go. Xenoestrogens like bisphenol A (BPA), bisphenol B (BPB), phthalates, etc. all build up over time with the use of plastics. If you are thinking ahead and preparing your food, chances are you are using plastic containers for your food and water. This problem is amplified if you like salty of acidic foods, as these foods really leach the toxins out.

Arsenic is another toxin that may be present in people doing their best to get healthy. If your diet program called for regular consumption of white rice, even small amounts such as ½ cup a day, you could have issues with this toxin. As I mentioned above, this toxin has been linked to insulin resistance and could be part of the reason you regained your weight so quickly after you ended your diet and exercise program, or even why you could not get the body you were after while doing the program.

You could have issues with mercury if you ate (or eat) a lot of canned fish, such as albacore tuna. If you have a leaky gut, as we discussed above, more toxins are likely to make their way into your system and affect you, especially in your compromised state following a high intensity program. You may need to detox to get better. Detoxification is the changing of toxic substances into non-toxic substances, so you can then transfer them out of the body in sweat, urine, and stool.

Toxins are interesting. You may have no problem with toxin A, until you encounter toxin B, or your body can no longer handle the toxin due to hormonal imbalance, stress, or other issues brought about by your diet and exercise plan.

Where you live, what you did as a past profession or do as a current profession, what your dad did in his past or present career, even the type of dental work you have had done, could cause toxins to build up. As you may be asking, "What does my mom or dad's profession have to do with my toxin exposure?" Let me give you a very real example. I have a client, a figure competitor, with a ton of medical issues that were really hard to pin down, as she has so many symptoms. Labs, overall, were normal, and we were having a tough time figuring her out. Finally, in our discussions of what to do next, I asked her that very question, "What did your dad do for a living?" Her response floored me, "He was a Round Up—glyphosate (N-(phosphonomethyl)glycine)—salesman and spent all day spray-ing weeds for clients." Glyphosate is one of the most toxic substances known to man—why it is approved for use anywhere near humans or other living animals is beyond me. Her father had been coming home from work every day with the poison all over him. Hugging and kissing his little girl every day after work, exposed her to high amounts of this toxin and, over time, her little body could not han-dle it. And now, twenty years later, she was still having issues with it. As we started to focus her recovery based on this fact, she started getting better.

There are several ways of measuring toxins in your body—blood tests, urine tests, hair tests, etc. If you are concerned you may have some, or are having a hard time recovering for whatever reason, find a good environmental doctor to run tests, and then help you clear the toxins that might be causing an issue.

Supporting the detox system would include removing the offending agents such as stopping your overexercising and undereating, looking for and then treating chronic infections, heavy metal or other possible toxic exposures in your past, including mold exposure.

Treating the body includes, but is not limited to: getting on the correct eating plan for your body, keeping your Ph above 6.5, ensuring you have a healthy liver and kidneys, correcting your hor-mones, including brain neurotransmitters, making sure you are on the correct supplements (particularly minerals), drinking plenty of clean water, sitting in a infrared sauna a few times a week, utilizing emotional or counseling support if relationship issues are at hand, and getting chelation therapy if it is indicated.

## At Home Labs

There are some absolutely wonderful tests you can do for/on yourself, without a doctor's order, to help you dial in your health and/or see if your Fat to Fit program has caused some issues. There are several tests one can do at home, but let me focus on what I consider the top six home tests and a quick interpretation of each:

## Fasting glucose

This test should be done first thing in the morning before you eat. Run to your local drug store and purchase a glucometer—a blood sugar reader. They are cheap and easy to use: a simple finger prick and a few minutes later, a number. This number should be between 70 and 84 for optimal health, less risk of cardiac disease, etc. If it is between 85 and 99, you are at risk for cardiac disease and diabetes, and will have a harder time losing fat. If your number is greater than 100, you are insulin resistant and we need to talk.

## One-Hour Post-prandial Glucose

Using the glucometer mentioned above, eat a "regular" meal by your standards, wait one hour and test your blood sugars. If your blood sugar is greater than 140 one hour after you eat, there are four things you need to do:

1. Cut back your carbs and/or increase your protein when you eat
2. Cut down on the amount of food you "regularly" eat
3. Read and apply the *RecoverMe* section below
4. See your doctor for treatment of insulin resistance, as this is impeding your ability to optimize your body.

## pH

This test starts by purchasing a pH strip from your local pharmacy or online (a good one is called hydrion S/R paper). A low urinary or salivary pH is indicative of insulin resistance, high levels of visceral fat, and high blood pressure. pH of both urine and saliva should be 6.5 to 6.8. If you have a pH less than that, you will find it hard to recover from your high exercise and low calorie program. You also will not detox your body very well if your pH is less than 6.5. If you plan to use a detox diet or cleanse, you must make sure your pH is appropriate.

Increasing pH can be done by daily intake of minerals, magnesium being of the utmost importance, drinking lemon water, and eating a lot of vegetables with your proteins, etc.

## Pulse

Your resting pulse can be a valuable tool in assessing the degree of sympathetic tone in your body and the stress your body is under. I would suggest you check it when you first wake up, while lying in bed, and then randomly throughout the day. Resting pulses greater than 75 are an issue. To paraphrase an old Chinese proverb, "You are only given so many heartbeats in a life time…keep your pulse low!"

## Blood Pressure

Blood pressure is an easy thing to measure. You can buy an electronic device (get the one for your arm, not your wrist), go to any doctor's office and have the nice nurse check it, or many grocery stores also have stations available for testing. A blood pressure of 130/85+ or less than 100/60 may indicate an issue, and you should visit your doctor to make sure no other issues are at hand.

## Heart Rate Variability (HRV)

Heart rate variability (HRV) is a measure of the variation in time between heartbeats. Under healthy/normal circumstances, the time between heartbeats is not consistent—it varies with every beat. As a Fat to Fit program tends to raise stress levels and lessen recovery, this simple test is yet another way to gauge how you are doing.

Using a heart rate monitor or smart phone app, measure how much variability there is between beats. If you have a high degree of HRV, you are in good shape and doing well. A low amount of variability reflects under-recovery and a stressed out, overtrained body.

## Medical Evaluation Conclusion

I have covered the more traditional labs in this brief review. Traditional labs do not always work, so many times we must use non-traditional methods to determine the real state of chaos your body is in. There are so many possibilities, based on each unique individual, I cannot cover them all, but I will quickly mention a few, as they are wonderful, but something only a very experienced pro-vider should test and interpret.

- Measuring one's anabolic to catabolic ratio.
    - 0 Anabolic means growth, repair and healing, and catabolic means break down or destruction. Undereating and overexercising tend to put you into a catabolic state—the degree of which is unique to the individual. Knowing that degree can help dictate the degree of aggressiveness in treatment. My favorite test for such things is to look at urinary metabolites of hormones over 24 hours. Yes—this means you collect your urine in a bucket over 24 hours. This measures

the 17 ketosteroids (anabolic) to 17 hydroxysteroids (catabolic) ratio.

- 28-day hormone tests for women

    o This is a salivary hormone test that looks at a full month of the primary hormones including estradiol, progesterone, testosterone, DHEA, cortisol, and melatonin. It is done by spitting in a little bottle 11 days of the month on a provided schedule. It affords not only a hormone curve and comparison of all of these hormones, but also a ratio of them for further insight into any potential concerns. False highs and lows such as those that occur with fat issues or thyroid dysfunction are avoided. It should only be used in women who are still menstruating or women who *should* be menstruating but stopped with their hypothetical health and body-obtaining program.

- Urinary hormone metabolites

    o This is a 24-hour urine test that looks at hormone metabolism. Once again, you must set aside time and space for some mild inconvenience—you must collect your urine in a bucket over 24 hours. Conventional testing, as mentioned above, only shows the parent hormones. Metabolites of hormones are essential to understand, as they show the degree of anabolic to catabolic metabolism, including inflammatory metabolites that affect quality of life and disease states or potentials (mentioned above). This can/could be of great benefit if you are having difficulty with your hormones.

- Genetic Testing

0 Your genetics certainly play a role in your ability to obtain that optimal physique. You can have genetic testing done to see your genetic potential for fat loss via diet and exercise. Genetic testing can look at your protein, fat, and carb utilization (what diet is best for you based on genetics). It can gauge how you lose fat in response to cardio training and your body composition response to weight training. It can look at intrinsic motivation to exercise, addictive behavior and stimulus control, and fitness response to cardio (why some people can run a marathon and others, with the same training, cannot). It can also look at your insulin sensitivity response to cardio training. Genetic testing is fun to see, but your lifestyle or epigenetics (above genetics) are still what matter most. You, based on your genetics, may never be a fitness super star like the bodybuilder Jay Cutler, or the fitness pro and Internet sensations, Steve Cook or Megan Thomas and Jamie Eason, but you can be in darn good shape, look great, and feel even better with your lifestyle! Daily things you do for the best body YOU can have. Let me give you a personal example: based on testing, my genetics are not very good for having a good physique, yet by most people's standards, I have one. Not thanks to my parents (nothing personal Mom and Dad), but because my *lifestyle* has allowed me to be at the top of **my** game, all the time—not just for a physique show!

o The other issue to consider with genetics, while we are on the subject, is the fact that it is not always the genetics you think are at play when it comes to a long-lasting body and health. Can some people stay thin forever, no matter what they do? The answer to that is yes. Besides not being fair, what can you think of that could be the reason they can do it? These fine people actually have great genetics for clearing toxins and/or they live in an environment that limits exposure to toxins. Something very hard to do nowadays. Thus our obesity problem and the popular false hope of a solution through a modern diet and exercise program.

- Advanced Lipid Testing

    0  I assume most of you reading this have had your cholesterol checked. This is basic lipid testing. Your high-density lipoprotein (HDL) or good cholesterol and your low-density lipoprotein (LDL) or bad cholesterol are important risk modification factors for your heart and total health. A low HDL and high LDL are indicative of greater cardiac risk, obesity, and diabetes, and are commonly seen following a Fat to Fit program.

    0  Advanced lipid testing allows your doctor to check very sensitive inflammatory markers, and several other cholesterol markers that are not only important for your health, but can also be used to fix your physique. How you eat obviously affects your health and knowing how to eat for your body is essential in recovering from your diet and exercise program. Beyond a doubt it is not the food you eat; it's what your body *does* with the food you eat! Advanced Lipid testing can be used to help dial that in with a little more accuracy. Markers include sdLDL (more detail below), LDL-P, HDL2b, oxidized LDL, Lp(a), TMAO, and an Omega-3 Index.

- **sdLDL**: The total LDL and HDL numbers are important, but they only tell part of the chronicle. Just as on the bodybuilding stage, size matters! Large, buoyant LDL particles are not dangerous; it's the small dense LDL particles that wreak havoc to your heart and vessels. Measuring these particles in the blood not only tells of cardiac risk, but also what your liver is doing with the food you eat. Someone with a high count of small LDL particles, called sdLDL, processes carbohydrates differently or eats too many carbohydrates for his/her body to handle. When a bodybuilder comes to me for a diet consult, I run this biomarker in part to see how many carbohydrates they are eating and how their body is processing them (not to mention I care about their total cardiac risk). High sdLDL counts can be indicative of too many carbohydrates for their body. Low sdLDL counts mean that their current diet is adequate, and I can start playing with their foods from there. Of course, some of this is genetically related, so I also check something called an apolipoprotein E genotype. This is a genetic test to help interpret the bio-markers with more individual accuracy. Studies have shown that certain people who eat a low fat/high carbohydrate diet induce a shift from large to small LDL particles, whereas low carbohydrate, high fat diets lower sdLDL and increase large LDL. Using the biomarker sdLDL, I can dial a person's eating plan to perfection. For someone with a high sdLDL when we first meet, I cut or change the carbs in their eating plan. Along with tracking their lean and fat mass, I recheck the lab after a few weeks to see what effect the diet change has had on the lab value. Most importantly, through this process, we are able to lower cardiac risk. But I have also found that when we learn the right proportion of carbs to fat in the diet via bio-markers, body goals can also be met. This is confirmed when I meet a person with an amazing physique who has everything dialed in: their sdLDL is perfect! For an older/wiser person who has been stuck at a weight or a look for some time, we can assist with some lean mass gain and fat loss beyond their previous expectations using this biomarker. For people recovering from a hard wear and tear diet and exercise program or just wanting to look good, this biomarker is an excellent way to help them avoid all the trial and error that goes into physique optimization!

Hopefully, this chapter has provided you with a starting point to talk with your doctor if you're chronically dieting, getting ready for a physique show, or you just feel lousy and want some answers. The next section, although shorter than the rest of the book, is the meat of the book. Now that you understand why you feel the way you do, and what labs can be done to help you dial in a response to the way you feel, we will talk about what to do about it!

# CHAPTER 9
## *RecoverMe* Exercise

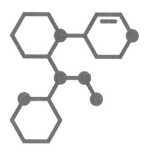

In this chapter, I will focus on the **RecoverMe** program using healthy or adequate exercise, and what to do around exercise with the pre- and post-workout meals.

Before we get into the **RecoverMe** exercise program, let me sum it up so as you are reading it makes sense: To recover from your Fat to Fit program, you must start with a good, homemade, stimulant free, pre-workout meal. You must follow the suggestions I will make concerning the post workout meal, as well. Exercise, whatever you decide on doing, must apply these following rules:

- When to exercise
    - ✓ First thing A.M. is ideal, but make it work for your schedule

- Amount of time exercising
  - ✓ Don't exceed 40 min a session
  - ✓ Ideally 20–30 minutes a session
- Number of days a week to exercise
  - ✓ 2 or 3 days a week for recovery (can increase later once you are healed)
- Number of days of rest between exercise
  - ✓ Allow your body to recover for at least one if not two days between exercise sessions
- Multiple training regimens
  - ✓ Change up what you do frequently
- Types of exercise
  - ✓ MIRTT (explained below)
  - ✓ Resistance training
  - ✓ Cardio or speed your heart rate up training
    - Not to exceed 65% max heart rate
  - ✓ Stretching
  - ✓ Pilates or Yoga
- Proper exercise monitoring
  - ✓ Keep your heart rate between 60% and 65% max heart rate for the training
  - ✓ Have your doctor run labs to make sure you are recovering

To put it in paragraph form: Exercise when it best fits your schedule (ideally first thing in the morning), two or three days a week, with one or two days of rest between, doing a variety of exercise types, using a combination of resistance training, stretching, and cardio while keeping your heart rate at 60% to 65% max. Don't exceed this, don't undercut this. Period. Trust me, you can increase the amount you do once you have fixed yourself.

## The *RecoverMe* Exercise Plan

Reading problem #1 in Chapter 4, you may have gotten the impression that exercise is bad. That is not the case. Too much exercise, without proper recovery is bad. Exercise is good. Do I sound like Tarzan? "Too much exercise…bad; recovery exercise…good."

If you are an enduring, hard-core, exercise freak, you are likely addicted to exercise. If I told you to quit it on the spot, you would roll your eyes, turn your back, and keep doing it. I hope to provide you with some programs/plans that will help you recover from the overexercising, undereating cycle you're in, so you can still feed the addiction, but get better in the process.

I am going to give you two things in this section: first and foremost, how to recover properly with/from exercise. Secondly, I am going to provide you with a few examples of programs that will work to help you heal. They will keep you fit, help you recover, make your relationship to exercise better, and have a healthy, long-lasting effect on your body.

In Chapter 4, Problem 1, we discussed how the exercise suggested by most exercise program beats the crap out of your body, due to the extremes of stress and the resulting cortisol and hormonal, inflammatory, metabolic, emotional, and mental effects that follow. The common thought with exercise these days is "more is better." That's classic alcoholic thinking. I have never seen anyone get a DUI after training hard, but I have seen plenty of people get incredibly dizzy and pass out from it. Here is another email, just received, describing that very fact:

*Hey Doc!*

*Hey, I am in a bit of a pickle here. I am headed on vacation with my family. I have been battling some of the same issues that brought me to my OBGYN after having my 3rd baby 2 years ago. I am having the same spells of dizziness. I wouldn't even call it that, as much as my equilibrium is just funky. It happens so randomly that I can't even pinpoint a cause. I have been training really hard at the gym and I will randomly get it there and I have to stop, close my eyes, and tell my brain that I promise the ground is not slanted and the floor isn't as close as my eyes are telling me. I have always had soft hair and it is coarse and falling out. I have always had a regular menstrual cycle of 28-30 days and my last cycle came 10 days early and the one before that 8 days early. I have been trying to get my body fat below 18% and have been following a healthy diet to get myself more toned and fit and nothing is happening. No matter what I eat, my body fat is slowly creeping back up. I lost from 26% down to 17% and was doing so well and then boom! Vertigo stuff hits again and no weight loss. I have been taking the supplements that we talked about to help manage stress, but I am at a loss here. I don't know what is going on, but I just want to go on vacation and enjoy spending time with my kiddos without feeling like I am going to tip over. Any ideas? and should I maybe check my thyroid levels again? Thank you so much for your help!!!*

Now going from 26% to 17% body fat is admirable, but if recovery is not there, not only does the progress stop, it screeches to a halt, turns around and readily goes the other way. And you do not feel good at the same time. The common viewpoint would make this girl exercise *more* to get the results to kick in again. The focus should be on recovery, meaning *less* exercise, a proper workup, and readjustment of diet and supplements. When I suggested this, she never responded. Very typical of someone influenced and fooled by the current thinking in the diet and exercise world.

## The Under-Recovery Syndrome

It is arguable that many professional athletes need to exercise a lot—hours upon hours a day. This is most certainly true, and ignoring their gifted genetics, as we discussed above, they also have something else to their benefit: They know how to recover.

I do not believe in what has been termed "The Overtraining Syndrome" as, again, if your job depended on it, you would exercise, move, work, whatever's necessary to make sure your kids are fed, and your personal goals are met. I don't think you can overtrain, but you can most certainly **under-recover**.

I call it the **Under-Recovery Syndrome** when exercise outdoes the body's ability to heal. If you do not recover as you should, the wear and tear on the body and brain eventually catches up to you. As you recall from above, the constant, purposeful, over activity of the metabolic, hormonal, and stress systems of the body, without proper recovery, eventually gets into lingering activation of this same system. Exercise, in particular, is hard on the body as it is purposeful, repetitive, intense activation of the brain, muscles, hormones, emotions, thoughts, and every other system you can think of. Once you are in this cycle and your stress system fails to shut down when you're not exercising, you start to crave the exercise and the endorphins released from it. It is a terribly vicious cycle some people get themselves into.

Would it be ideal to break this cycle by stopping the exercise and resting? Yes, it would. But let us be realistic—most people, after doing a Fat to Fit program, have a hard time stopping. Like I said—it is addicting. So what is the solution?

The solution is to continue exercising in a "keep you out of the chronic overactivation cycle" and then make sure you are recovering properly.

## How to Recover from Exercise

Recovery from excessive exercise is not just in what you do following the exercise. Recovery happens all the time you are not exercising. What you do with your time outside the gym dictates your ability to recover in the gym. We will get into that in a lot more detail in the following chapters on eating, supplements, and sleep. In this section, I will briefly review anabolic steroids and the pre- and post-workout meals.

## Anabolic/Androgenic Steroids (AAS)

Let me quickly review anabolic steroids, as this is **not** the way I suggest recovering, and then detail the rest as part of your *RecoverMe* program:

I mentioned anabolic androgenic steroids (AAS) earlier, as they are used by a growing number of individuals to help recover from their diet and exercise program, are part of the problem. I feel it is important to outline some details about AAS, so you understand how they work, and how the *RecoverMe* program in this book does basically the same thing without the side effects or problems associated with the drugs.

Most AAS are hormones. Hormones are messengers that regulate growth, alter body mass, direct reproduction, control behavior, regulate minerals in the body, etc. Anabolic steroids are a group of hormones created to duplicate the beneficial aspects of testosterone.

When dealing specifically with muscle cells, AAS tell the muscle cells to increase protein synthesis, which allows the muscle to grow faster, recover quicker, etc., increase creatine phosphate synthesis, the substrate needed for energy (i.e., makes you stronger), increase the storage of glycogen in the muscle cell, which increases the cell's size by the amount of glycogen and by the accompanying water that comes with it, and increase nutrient uptake by the cell.

These activities of AAS equate to one thing: recovery. That is the secret to AAS—recovery. AAS help you recover from the extremes of exercise and dieting and, therefore, you get the increased muscle growth, fat burning, etc.

That is the shortest, most concise, summary of AAS I could come up with, so let's delve into the importance of the other modes of recovery. Keep in mind a few of the key points above, as they will come up again when discussing alternative/better ways to recover:

## Pre- and Post-Workout Meals

Almost all of the current diet and exercise programs out there suggest pre- and post-workout meals. My book, **Better Than Steroids,** written over 12 years ago, really brought these two meals to the forefront of the physique world. Many of the pre-workout meals/supplements out there are part of the concern, with all the stimulants involved. As your body is in complete disarray following a modern suggested diet and exercise program, I would like to suggest some new ideas for pre- and post-workout meals that fall into the *RecoverMe* lifestyle.

Before we get into that, let's briefly review what both a pre- and post-workout meal does or should do.

A good pre-workout meal ramps up energy stores for your workout, and should decrease the catabolic hormone, cortisol, by causing a slight rise in insulin. It needs to lessen muscle damage and inflammation with the proper antioxidants and anti-inflammatories, and basically set the ground work for quicker recovery following your workout.

A good post-workout meal helps repair muscles by supplying the proper and adequate nutrients, thereby decreasing muscle damage and accelerating repair and recovery. It should increase protein synthesis and replenish glycogen stores in the muscle, and increase Nitric Oxide (NO) synthesis, thereby increasing blood flow. When the right ingredients are in place, fat oxidation increases, thereby burning more fat. It should also help the body in the removal of waste products, such as lactic acid, and replenish energy stores, such as creatine phosphate.

Now that you understand the importance of your pre- and post-workout meal, even though your exercise intensity may be changing a little—see below—let's design one specifically for you and your *RecoverMe* program:

## Pre-Workout Meal

The pre-workout meal in a *RecoverMe* program needs to consist of a few precise ingredients that specifically target the needs of someone while doing or after an intense diet and exercise program. We need to think in terms of appropriate hormone stimulators, good antioxidants, and specific herbs/vitamins/minerals that can be utilized for specific concerns of a Fat to Fit survivor.

The pre-workout meal in a *RecoverMe* program is ideally made by you. I have designed one that hits the mark for most people if you are interested, but ideally I would encourage you to mix and match the ingredients listed below to fit **YOUR** specific need(s), based on your symptoms, and the workup you and your doctor did together, as outlined in Chapter 8.

After each potential ingredient, I have listed why this particular ingredient may be of special benefit to you. I would suggest you find all of these in powder form, or at least in capsule form (to break open), so you can dump the suggested dose into your pre-workout drink.

## Pre-workout Meal Hormone Stimulators

This is the "food" part of a pre-workout meal. The dose of "food" does not have to be, and should not, be a lot. Save the energy for a good meal. Food causes the change in hormones needed for recovery and repair. This would include a protein source and a carb source. The types of protein and carbs you choose are based on how you are feeling and any symptoms you are experiencing, as well as the testing you may have done with your doctor. For example; if you did the food allergy testing mentioned above and found you had an intolerance to milk products (as many, if not most people do after three whey protein drinks a day), you may want to consider a pea of hemp based protein powder.

## Protein Source (dose: 10-15 grams):

- High-grade whey protein
    - If you have no allergies or concerns with milk products
- Pea-based protein powder
    - Pea-based protein is a whole protein almost identical to whey based protein as far as macronutrients and the amount of branch chain amino acids (BCAA).
    - Use if you have been using whey-based protein forever or, if you feel you may have some mild concerns with milk products (such as bloating, sinus issues, etc.), switch to a pea-based protein,

or use it intermittently to give your body a break from milk products.

- Bonito Proteins

    - Use if you have high blood pressure or anxiety issues

    - Bonito (*Sarda orientalis*) is a fish belonging to the tuna and mackerel family and that is traditionally consumed in Japan. Bonito peptides provide safe, natural blood pressure support for individuals who may be having blood pressure issues, especially with all the stimulants used in a Fat to Fit Program. Bonito peptides have been shown to inhibit ACE activity. ACE inhibitors are a favorite drug in a doctor's blood pressure lowering regimen, as they are effective and very safe. An example of an ACE inhibitor drug is Lisinopril.

## Carbohydrate Source (dose: 5-10 grams):

- D-ribose

    - Use this simple carbohydrate, as it is the best overall source of a pre-workout carbohydrate in a ***RecoverMe*** process following a Fat to Fit program.

    - You will find a lot of information on D-ribose, in regard to heart disease and heart health. You will also hear of its use in chronic fatigue syndrome and fibromyalgia. As many survivors of a popular diet and exercise programs have similar symptoms, D-ribose is the carbohydrate of choice. It is a simple sugar that improves lactate disposal (waste products) built up with exercise/muscle use, by transporting lactate back into energy cycle. It also improves ATP (energy) production and improves production of glutathione (one of the strongest antioxidants known to man).

0 Add creatine, in a dose of 5 grams, to optimize D-ribose

- Resistant Starch

    - Resistant starch is basically a carbohydrate that is not absorbed very well. It will have some mild hormonal effects, but its importance in your **RecoverMe** program is in reducing pH levels, feeding the friendly bacteria in your gut, and indirectly feeding the cells in your gut by increasing the amount of butyrate.

    - A great example is banana flour from green bananas, raw potatoes, and a whole variety of premade selections or ones you can do yourself.

## Antioxidants and Minerals–Dose Listed Following Each One

- Vitamin C

    - Dose: 500 to 2500 mg

    - Vitamin C has so many beneficial properties and uses, I will not even attempt to cover them here. Full books have been written on the topic, with thousands of medically reviewed articles. Simply said: you need it!

- At higher doses, it may cause some stomach irritation and loose stools, so go slowly with it if you are not used to it.

- Mixed Tocotrienols/Tocopherols (Vitamin E)
    - Dose: 1 gel cap (400–800 IU) with pre-workout meal
    - Vitamin E is composed of eight different compounds—four tocopherols (the most common form of vitamin E) and four others, known as tocotrienols. This vitamin does many things in the body including, but not limited to: neuroprotection, acting as an antioxidant, improving glucose and insulin tolerance, and acting as an anti-inflammatory.
    - It is a fat-soluble vitamin, so be sure to get it in a gel/oil capsule so it gets absorbed correctly.

- Magnesium
    - Dose: 100 mg (elemental magnesium)
    - Magnesium is involved in or necessary for over 300 different metabolic activities in the body including: integral in ATP production, oxygen uptake, central nervous system function, electrolyte balance, glucose metabolism, muscle function, heart rate and function, bone density, etc.
    - Exercise, especially at the Fat to Fit intensity, significantly depletes magnesium. It is part of

the reason so many patients come to me with muscle tightness and a tendency to pull or get injured easily. It also shows up as severe muscle fatigue, reduced stamina, and nervousness.

- Magnesium is a mineral you need to take throughout the day to ensure adequate amounts in your cells.

- As I mentioned in Chapter 8, you need to follow your magnesium levels with your doctor on a regular basis while doing or following any intense diet and exercise program using a RBC Mg+ level.

## Other Important Ingredients

- Taurine

    - Dose: 3 grams

    - Taurine is an amino acid that has some central alpha agonist activity. It helps slow down the sympathetic nervous system and, thereby, helps control heart rate, anxiety, etc.

- Hawthorn Berry

    - Dose: 200 mg

    - Most of the supplements out there are higher doses, so use a capsule form and dump just part of it into your pre-workout meal. Save the rest for later.

    - Hawthorn berry acts as a beta-blocker. Like taurine, it helps to limit heart rate, so you can finish your exercise session without your heart rate getting too high and causing further issues. It also helps control the high blood pressure response people tend to have both with and following a lot of the diet and exercise programs out there.

- Find a supplement containing *Crataegus oxyacantha*, which is standardized (1.8% strength) to contain the flavonoid vitexin.

- Acetyl-L-Carnitine
    - Dose: 1000–3000 mg
    - Acetyl-L-Carnitine is an amino acid that does several things in the body. It basically allows different tissues, especially brain and muscle tissue, to produce energy. It supports the normal breakdown of free, long chain, fatty acids for transport to and oxidation in the mitochondria.

- Beta-alanine
    - Dose: 1000–3000 mg
    - Beta-alanine is a non-essential amino acid that can be found in almost all premade workout drinks. Studies have shown it to be a metabolically active substance that can improve athletic performance. Supplementation with β-alanine has been shown to increase the concentration of carnosine in muscles, which in turn decreases fatigue and increases the ability of the muscles to work effectively.

- It is very common for this supplement to cause reflux or "acid indigestion." If this occurs, back off on the dose and slowly increase it.

- Green tea

    - Dose: Two tea bags

    - Green tea (*Camelia sinensis*) is an abundant source of antioxidants, notably epigallocatechin gallate (EGCG), a polyphenol. Polyphenols combat oxidative stress and act as anti-inflammatories. That simply means first, that it is really good for you, and second, it has been shown to increase energy and improve results from exercise, when used prior to exercising. One study that had participants exercise on a bike, one hour at a time, three times a week for four weeks, showed a 25% increase in fat oxidation and a body fat decrease of 1.63%, compared to placebo. Exercise performance also improved by 10.9% in the green tea group.

    - You could also empty a 640-mg polyphenol capsule into your pre-workout meal if you would rather not drink tea before exercise.

- Beetroot

    - Dose: 500 mL of standard beetroot or 1000 mg of powder

    - Studies have shown beetroot juice increases blood flow to the skeletal muscles by 38% during exercise. Research has also shown that beetroot juice improves brain function. As brain function is compromised by over intense diet and exercise programs, this is a wonderful addition to a pre-workout meal, as *appropriate* exercise also improves brain function. Beets are loaded with dietary nitrate, which is converted to nitrites and then to nitric oxide after consumption. Nitric oxide boosts exercise performance by increasing oxygen availability to exercising muscles via increased blood flow. As the brain is a prevailing utilizer of oxygen and directs blood flow/oxygen to parts of the body in need, beetroot juice plus exercise greatly strengthens an area of the brain called the somatomotor cortex.

## Post-Workout Meal

During exercise, even the moderate exercise described below, energy stores are depleted. This includes ATP and creatine phosphate (CP). Muscle glycogen stores are drained and catabolic hormones, such as cortisol, epinephrine, and norepinephrine, are elevated. These all break down muscle in an already depleted body! Free radicals are generated by the exercise and an inflammatory response occurs. As if your body has not been through enough! The post-workout meal will prevent further destruction of your body, via the following mechanisms:

- Decreases muscle damage, thereby increasing muscle mass
- Accelerates repair and recovery
- Replenishes glycogen stores in the muscle
- Increases Nitric Oxide (NO) synthesis, thereby increasing blood flow

- Increases fat oxidation, burning more fat
- Increases protein synthesis
- Increases removal of waste products such as lactic acid
- Replenishes energy stores such as creatine phosphate

The post-workout meal in a *RecoverMe* program is a little more generalized and, therefore, not as tedious. Some particular supplements are needed, however, under certain conditions, as I have listed below. Again, we need to think in terms of appropriate hormone stimulators, good antioxidants, and specific herbs/vitamins/minerals that can be utilized for specific concerns of a Fat to Fit survivor.

## Post-workout meal hormone stimulators

This is similar to the pre-workout meal above, other than the carbohydrate source.

## Protein source (dose: 15-20 grams):

- High-grade whey protein
    - If you have no allergies or concerns with milk products
- Pea or hemp based protein powder
    - Use if you have mild concerns, or use intermittently to give your body a break from the milk products.
- Bonito Proteins
    - Use if you have high blood pressure or anxiety issues

## Carbohydrate source (dose: 10-15 grams):

- Resistant Starch as mentioned above
    - Following exercise, it lowers LPS and helps modify IL-6
- D-Ribose as mentioned above
- Simple table sugar may have a role here, in very small amounts, as it certainly causes the hormonal response we want following an exercise routine.
    - Not only is it cheap, but very accessible

## Other important ingredients

- Holy Basil 400 mg
    - Holy Basil (*Ocimum sanctum*) is a member of the mint, or *labiatae*, family. It is closely related to the sweet basil (*Ocimum basilicum*) frequently used in cooking.
    - Holy Basil dampens the cortisol response caused by exercise. It is also a good antioxidant and anti-inflammatory.
- CoQ10 30–60 mg
    - CoQ10 is naturally made in the body; therefore, it is not classified as a vitamin. There have been multiple studies on it, concerning cardiac health, blood pressure, etc., but it also has some studies of its use to reduce muscle damage from exercise.

- It does a lot of its work in the mitochondria of the cells, and helps supply the body with energy in the form of Adenosine Triphosphate or ATP.
- Vitamin C, Vitamin E, and magnesium, as mentioned above.

## *RecoverMe* Exercise Programs

Having, at one time or other, followed a hardcore undereating and overexercising plan, you fall into one of two categories: 1. I will never exercise again! Or, 2. I want to keep doing hardcore, intense exercise!

If you are a #1, please start moving again. Your *RecoverMe* program depends on it! You must move to rebalance and shift hormones back to the way they should be. Movement is essential with the prescribed eating plans and supplements below. This is not a Fat to Fit program—this one does not come with false promises, nor will it interrupt your schedule, and make you feel bad in the long run. Movement is as important as any drug, supplement, or diet I could prescribe for you in your road to *RecoverMe*. Trust me. The exercise plans listed below are self-graduated, so start slow and progress slowly. If you would rather not participate in a planned activity, I would encourage some form of simple movement, such as walking or hiking, and a resistance training program, like *8 to Won* listed below.

For you #2s out there—stay within the lines drawn here! You have an unhealthy relationship with exercise. You can come to my OEA (Over Exercisers Anonymous) classes with me (I am now a sponsor). Most people can exercise as they wish as long as they are following the prescribed diet and supplement program and are using the medications or hormones prescribed by their doctor. That is part of the reason this book provides a package for you to follow. Part of your exercise issue is because it makes you feel good. It is the only time your endorphins and other fun brain chemicals are flowing, when you are suffering the effects of your diet and exercise program. Getting the correct diagnosis with the work up I described, optimizing your hormone and nutrient status, removing any potential toxins, getting your gut to work correctly—all these things will make your exercise usage tolerable. You will enjoy your exercise again, not just feel like you have to do it!

The easiest thing for you regular exercisers out there to do, or just you people who enjoy exercise, is to continue what you are doing, just cut way back on the intensity. I would encourage you to follow the recommendations listed directly below, and incorporate them into a program you enjoy.

I will suggest a few simple exercise programs for you to follow or at least try, but before I do, let us talk about some very important specifics of the exercise programs (the ones below or yours) to be used to help you **RecoverMe**.

## When to Exercise

Ideally, exercise is done first thing in the morning, when you wake up. Metabolically, physiologically, and for circadian reasons, especially recovering from an concentrated diet and exercise pro-gram, this is important. As you now know, your brain neurotrans-mitters, thyroid, sex hormones and adrenal hormones are off. Your body literally does not know night from day, as everything got so out of whack following that silly program. Exercising in the morning, along with other modalities I have and will mention, is a way to start setting things right again.

In reality, the best time to exercise is *when you can!* It has to fit your lifestyle. You already threw a wrench into your lifestyle doing the Fat to Fit program, so be a little more flexible and kinder to your-self. If trying to get your exercise in stresses you out, you are getting an F in your **RecoverMe** program. Make sense?

As we are slaves to our calendars, put your exercise plans on your smart phone, Google calendar, or old-fashioned wall calendar with the pretty pictures of flowers or funny animals on it. You must write them down or you won't do them. Have you ever missed an appointment because you forgot to write it down? Yeah, me too. Write it down.

## The Amount of Time Exercising

This one can be debated pretty seriously, but I don't care—I know what works for people recovering from overexercising and undereating. You should not exercise for more than 40 minutes per session. Ideally, you go for 20 to 30 minutes a session. That is it. Go longer, especially in the recovery phase, and you start to impact your hormones in a negative way. Do you know what that means? It means you don't get better.

## The Number of Days Per Week to Exercise

"Authorities" and "experts" out there give all sorts of recommendations for exercise. The difficulty with these so-called experts is they all come from different areas of expertise. The heart health experts tell you to exercise X many days a week. Weight loss gurus tell you Y many times a week. Your personal trainer, who makes more per hour than you do, tells you to do it daily—for obvious reasons. So, that being said, please allow me to be an expert in your *RecoverMe* program: You should exercise two to three days a week. Once again, that's it. Remember our goal here. Once you have mastered *RecoveredMe*, your frequency can increase.

## The Number of Days to Rest between Exercise Days

So, you ask, does that mean I should exercise for 30 minutes Monday, Tuesday, and Wednesday, and take the rest of the week off?

Well, honestly, if that is what your schedule allows, then yes! Don't increase your cortisol trying to work out little details like this. A Monday, Wednesday, Saturday schedule might be better for your little body, so you can **RecoverMe** between exercise sessions, but focus on making it fit your current schedule.

## Multiple Training Regimens

You need to figure out several different things you like to do. However, you must include the following:

- Resistance training
    - Using inanimate objects, with handles that do not fight back. Your local gym will work. Body weight exercises like those with MIRTT (described below) also work. Exercising on the space station does not work—no gravity.
- Heart rate raising activity
    - A walk or light jog, riding a bike (not racing a bike), going for a hike, etc.
- Stretching
    - Pilates or Yoga, or just sitting on the floor and stretching after a hot shower or sauna. If you don't know how to stretch, there are plenty of resources online.
- At least one outside activity each week
    - This one is a must! You should do an exercise activity outside if your situation allows it. Tree huggers like me have always found great relief and comfort in nature. Exposure to real sunlight

increases the brain hormone serotonin and makes you feel good! Intuitively, we know that peace and tranquility are in the multiple colors and sounds available. My favorite place to relax and actually feel some peace is outside, watching and listening to all that nature has to offer. Science supports this fact. It seems that brain connectivity, when listening to man-made (artificial) sounds, shows an internally-directed attention focus similar to that seen when the brain is under attack via anxiety, posttraumatic stress disorder, and/or depression. However, when it hears sounds of nature such as birds chirping, a bubbling brook, a waterfall, wind through the trees, or the rustle of an Aspen, the brain exhibits signs of outwardly-directed attention focus. This equates to brain and nervous system activity associated with relaxation and stress reduction. Studies have shown that those with the greatest amount of stress also found the greatest amount of stress relief with natural sounds. With it, make a change in your stress levels—get outside and enjoy nature's sounds and sights as often as possible.

## Types of Exercise

You need a good combination of resistance training and heart moving exercise. Ideally, you get both at once. Resistance training with weights or against gravity using your own body will work, but the pace should be brisk and get the ol' ticker ticking! It takes far too much time to spend 30 minutes weight training, then another

30 minutes riding a stair-stepper. I like the term MIRTT—moderate intensity resistance training techniques to describe the majority of the exercises I teach people wanting to get in shape, without the actual Fat to Fit program boo-boos. MIRTT incorporates resistance training, basically without rest periods between most prescribed exercises. The **Negative 5** program below, for example, has you do a set of 6 to 8 reps of push-ups, followed immediately by one leg chair squats, then towel rows, then jumping pull-ups, followed immediately by wall resisted lateral raises, and end with body hamstring curls. Then repeat that sequence one more time. Occasionally, through the series, check your heart rate really quickly to make sure you are maintaining 60% to 65% max. See below for examples.

## Proper Exercise Measurement Protocols

During exercise, you want to make sure you are not overdoing it—especially if you fall under #2 above. With the suggested type and examples of training, keep your heart rate between 60% and 65% max. Use the following equation:

220 – age multiplied by 0.60 and then again by .65 = suggested *RecoverMe* exercise heart rate

For example, if you are 35 years old,

220 – 35 = 185 × 0.60 (then do with 0.65) = 111 to 120 heart rate

This example would exercise to keep your heart rate between 111 and 120 beats per minute while training. Not lower, not higher—try to keep it there. If it goes higher, back off. If it is lower, pick up your pace a little.

Exercise assessment with *RecoverMe* training can also be done in the lab, via your doctor. Looking at a few measurements like 8OHDG, or other measures of oxidative stress, can be a good way to assess your efforts. Following lean and fat mass is also suggested. Avoid the scale unless you are using it with body composition. Scales lie—especially in recovery programs.

## *RecoverMe* Exercise Programs

I have literally thousands of exercise programs I could have added here. I have been a personal trainer, collecting exercise programs since the early 1980s, and I am a nerd, so I kept them all!

I narrowed it down to a few, as eventually we all find what we like to do on a regular basis. That is what you need to stick to in the long term—something you enjoy. These programs I listed here are sample programs for **RecoverMe**.

The **8 to Won** is the simplest program—for someone trying to lose weight, get moving again after an injury, or someone so burnt out on exercise from their Fat to Fit program, they swore they would never do it again. Try it—it is simple, but effective!

**Negative 5** is a more involved program that employs techniques that allow you to get in and out of your exercise clothes in a quick, timely manner. You can do it in the gym or at home. For you exercise minded people, you can add to, change, or modify any of the exercises to fit your needs.

**Speed Sets** is another version of *medium intensity resistance training technique* or MIRTT that is fun to do. As I suggest you do it no more than three days a week, it allows great results without over-doing it (if your **RecoverMe** program in total is on track!).

The **Full-Body CrossFit Program** is another MIRTT for people who like to be like Bruce Lee or Tarzan and throw their own bodies around. There are tons of options with this one, so go to my web site if you would like to see more (drwilley.com).

## *8 to Won*

8 to Won is a very simple MIRTT program. It is called 8 to Won because it has eight exercises in each session, and if you do all eight weeks, you've won! Really—it makes you feel a lot better even as simple as it is. It can be done at home, in your

office, in the bathroom—wherever. It's designed for you type 1s out there who really don't want to exercise. It can also be done by someone trying to break into the exercise arena or who is just trying to get healthy. I have had great luck using it with some of my wonderful fibromyalgia and chronic pain patients, as it is simple, requires no equipment, and is done quickly!

It is a progressive program, done three days a week, with gradual and incremental increases in the amount of time spent doing the exercises over the course of eight weeks.

Get some sort of timer clock to time yourself.

## Week 1

**1 minute intervals: 10 seconds doing the activity, 50 seconds rest (go on to the next activity and repeat 10 seconds exercise, 50 seconds rest)**

| | |
|---|---|
| 10 seconds | Jog/run in place |
| Rest 50 seconds | |
| 10 seconds | Jumping jacks |
| Rest 50 seconds | |
| 10 seconds | Cross-country skier |
| Rest 50 seconds | |
| 10 seconds | Push-ups off wall or desk |
| Rest 50 seconds | |
| 10 seconds | Squats |
| Rest 50 seconds | |
| 10 seconds | Lunges |
| Rest 50 seconds | |
| 10 seconds | Planks or crunches |
| Rest 50 seconds | |
| 10 seconds | Calf raises |

## Week 2

1 minute intervals: 15 seconds doing the activity, 45 seconds rest (go on to the next activity and repeat 15 seconds exercise, 45 seconds rest)

| | |
|---|---|
| 15 seconds | Jog/run in place |
| Rest 45 seconds | |
| 15 seconds | Jumping jacks |
| Rest 45 seconds | |
| 15 seconds | Cross-country skier |
| Rest 45 seconds | |
| 15 seconds | Push-ups off wall or desk |
| Rest 45 seconds | |
| 15 seconds | Squats |
| Rest 45 seconds | |
| 15 seconds | Lunges |
| Rest 45 seconds | |
| 15 seconds | Planks or crunches |
| Rest 45 seconds | |
| 15 seconds | Calf raises |

## Week 3

1 minute intervals: 20 seconds doing the activity, 40 seconds rest (go on to the next activity and repeat 20 seconds exercise, 40 seconds rest)

| | |
|---|---|
| 20 seconds | Jog/run in place |
| Rest 40 seconds | |
| 20 seconds | Jumping jacks |
| Rest 40 seconds | |
| 20 seconds | Cross-country skier |
| Rest 40 seconds | |
| 20 seconds | Push-ups off wall or desk |
| Rest 40 seconds | |
| 20 seconds | Squats |
| Rest 40 seconds | |
| 20 seconds | Lunges |
| Rest 40 seconds | |
| 20 seconds | Planks or crunches |
| Rest 40 seconds | |
| 20 seconds | Calf raises |

## Week 4

1 minute intervals: 25 seconds doing the activity, 35 seconds rest (go on to the next activity and repeat 25 seconds exercise, 35 seconds rest)

| | |
|---|---|
| 25 seconds | Jog/run in place |
| Rest 35 seconds | |
| 25 seconds | Jumping jacks |
| Rest 35 seconds | |
| 25 seconds | Cross-country skier |
| Rest 35 seconds | |
| 25 seconds | Push-ups off wall or desk |
| Rest 35 seconds | |
| 25 seconds | Squats |
| Rest 35 seconds | |
| 25 seconds | Lunges |
| Rest 35 seconds | |
| 25 seconds | Planks or crunches |
| Rest 35 seconds | |
| 25 seconds | Calf raises |

## Week 5

1 minute intervals: 30 seconds doing the activity, 30 seconds rest (go on to the next activity and repeat 30 seconds exercise, 30 seconds rest)

| | |
|---|---|
| 30 seconds | Jog/run in place |
| Rest 30 seconds | |
| 30 seconds | Jumping jacks |
| Rest 30 seconds | |
| 30 seconds | Cross-country skier |
| Rest 30 seconds | |
| 30 seconds | Push-ups off wall or desk |
| Rest 30 seconds | |
| 30 seconds | Squats |
| Rest 30 seconds | |
| 30 seconds | Lunges |
| Rest 30 seconds | |
| 30 seconds | Planks or crunches |
| Rest 30 seconds | |
| 30 seconds | Calf raises |

## Week 6

1 minute intervals: 35 seconds doing the activity, 25 seconds rest (go on to the next activity and repeat 35 seconds exercise, 25 seconds rest)

| | |
|---|---|
| 35 seconds | Jog/run in place |
| Rest 25 seconds | |
| 35 seconds | Jumping jacks |
| Rest 25 seconds | |
| 35 seconds | Cross-country skier |
| Rest 25 seconds | |
| 35 seconds | Push-ups off wall or desk |
| Rest 25 seconds | |
| 35 seconds | Squats |
| Rest 25 seconds | |
| 35 seconds | Lunges |
| Rest 25 seconds | |
| 35 seconds | Planks or crunches |
| Rest 25 seconds | |
| 35 seconds | Calf raises |

## Week 7

1 minute intervals: 40 seconds doing the activity, 20 seconds rest (go on to the next activity and repeat 40 seconds exercise, 20 seconds rest)

| | |
|---|---|
| 40 seconds | Jog/run in place |
| Rest 20 seconds | |
| 40 seconds | Jumping jacks |
| Rest 20 seconds | |
| 40 seconds | Cross-country skier |
| Rest 20 seconds | |
| 40 seconds | Push-ups off wall or desk |
| Rest 20 seconds | |
| 40 seconds | Squats |
| Rest 20 seconds | |
| 40 seconds | Lunges |
| Rest 20 seconds | |
| 40 seconds | Planks or crunches |
| Rest 20 seconds | |
| 40 seconds | Calf raises |

## Week 8

1 minute intervals: 45 seconds doing the activity, 15 seconds rest (go on to the next activity and repeat 45 seconds exercise, 15 seconds rest)

| | |
|---|---|
| 45 seconds | Jog/run in place |
| Rest 15 seconds | |
| 45 seconds | Jumping jacks |
| Rest 15 seconds | |
| 45 seconds | Cross-country skier |
| Rest 15 seconds | |
| 45 seconds | Push-ups off wall or desk |
| Rest 15 seconds | |
| 45 seconds | Squats |
| Rest 15 seconds | |
| 45 seconds | Lunges |
| Rest 15 seconds | |
| 45 seconds | Planks or crunches |
| Rest 15 seconds | |
| 45 seconds | Calf raises |

## Negative 5

*Negative 5* is a combination of concentric resistance training, with a focus on the eccentric or negative portion of the movement. Concentric contraction is a movement you picture when resistance training. For example: pushing the bar off your chest in a bench press type movement is the concentric portion of the movement. Lowering the bar back to your chest is the eccentric portion of the movement. Eccentric training focuses on slowing down the elongation or stretch of the muscle. It is also called "the negative" portion of the movement (hence the term negative in *Negative 5*). When one focuses on the eccentric portion of the movement, more muscle fibers are recruited and studies show that our bodies respond much quicker with an increase in strength, muscle size, muscle repair, and hormone balance—in particular, optimizing insulin and leptin at the level of the muscle. In other words, with training focused on the eccentric portion of the movement, you become more insulin-sensitive and leptin-sensitive. This is a hormonal absolute must if anyone hopes to find optimal hormone balance throughout their body (this would include proper thyroid function, proper brain function, proper adrenal gland function, and proper sex hormone function!. Since this optimizes hormones on all levels, the amount of time it takes is also much shorter! You no longer need to spend hours exercising, based on false information, to get results; as I have said for years and years and actually use to end all my published exercise articles—*TRAIN WITH YOUR BRAIN!*

*Negative 5* training is truly training smarter, not harder.

## How to Utilize a *Negative 5* Training System

As I mentioned earlier, *Negative 5* places focus on the eccentric portion of traditional compound (multiple muscle) movements. In essence, all of the eccentric or negative portions of the classic movements are done at a five-count pace. In other words, you do the positive or concentric portion of the movement at a normal speed, and the eccentric or negative portion of the movement utilizing a five count (o*ne Mississippi, two Mississippi, three Mississippi, four Mississippi, five Mississippi*), with a two-count pause in between the eccentric and concentric movement (*one Mississippi, two Mississippi*), and repeat the concentric portion of the movement at a normal speed.

Utilizing a bench press as an example:

From the starting position, with your arms extended, lower the bar to your chest using the five-count mentioned above. Pause on your chest for a two count, and press it back up at normal speed. Repeat.

As this is much more difficult than it sounds, I suggest doing 5 to 6 repetitions per set utilizing the weight you would normally exercise with. Please see the detailed exercise descriptions for some examples of sets and reps.

Eccentric contractile movements should be slow and controlled movements. I would encourage you to exercise with a partner to assist you with this style of training. Using lighter weight and using slow controlled movements are essential while your body is healing from the Fat to Fit program.

Eccentric contractions can cause a lot more muscle soreness, in particular delayed onset muscle soreness or DOMS, so go slowly with it. We are trying to get you better, not set you back a few months. DOMS will be minimized with the *Negative 5* training system as you only have to exercise two or three times a week to get hormonally optimal results.

## Getting Started:

### Types of exercises

*Negative 5* incorporates basic exercise movements that maximize muscle optimization (size, strength, shape) and contraction. This means we use more "compound" movements, or movements that utilize more than one muscle group. For example: a squat is a compound movement, as it utilizes the buttocks, hip abductors, hip adductors, quadriceps, hamstrings, and gastrocnemius (calves).

### Number/types of exercises

*Negative 5* utilizes the basic movements that train the most muscles, at the maximal intensity, in short durations. There are six basic movements in the *Negative 5* repertoire:

- ✓ an upper body press, with focus on chest, shoulders, and triceps
- ✓ a squat movement, with focus on the quadriceps and buttocks
- ✓ a row, with focus on the upper mid-back and biceps

- ✓ a pull-up, with focus on the upper outer back and biceps
- ✓ a lateral raise, with focus on the shoulders
- ✓ a hamstring curl, with focus on the hamstrings and calves

|  | Sunday | Monday | Tuesday | Wednesday | Thursday | Friday | Saturday |
|---|---|---|---|---|---|---|---|
| Upper body press |  | 2 sets of 6 to 8 reps |  |  | 2 sets of 6 to 8 reps |  |  |
| Squat |  | 2 sets of 6 to 8 reps |  |  | 2 sets of 6 to 8 reps |  |  |
| Row |  | 2 sets of 6 to 8 reps |  |  | 2 sets of 6 to 8 reps |  |  |
| Pull-up |  | 2 sets of 6 to 8 reps |  |  | 2 sets of 6 to 8 reps |  |  |
| Lateral raise |  | 2 sets of 6 to 8 reps |  |  | 2 sets of 6 to 8 reps |  |  |
| Hamstring curl |  | 2 sets of 6 to 8 reps |  |  | 2 sets of 6 to 8 reps |  |  |

## Sets and Reps

As *Negative 5* utilizes more muscle fibers than traditional exercise or resistance training, sets and reps can be kept to a minimum. This will also help DOMS especially when you're first getting started. *Negative 5* is two to three sets of 6 to 8 repetitions, per exercise, 2 to 3 times a week. Using the MIRTT, you do your upper body press, then immediately go to squats, and then to a row, and so on. Before you do them again, check your heart rate—if it is higher than your calculated 65%, slow down. If it is under your calculated 60%, speed up.

## Health Club or Home?

There are two types of training programs utilizing the *Negative 5* systems. The first includes exercises using machines, weights, and dumbbells performed in a health club or gym setting. For ease, I will call this training "Version 1." The second type of training is using body weight (yours and, if you want, your exercise partner's) that you can do at home or anywhere for that matter. We will call this training "Version 2."

**Version 1**

The gym version will utilize exercises you are likely very familiar with:

- an upper body press, with focus on chest, shoulders, and triceps
  - ✓ bench press or incline press
- a squat movement, with focus on the quadriceps and buttocks
  - ✓ a barbell or dumbbell squat, or a leg press machine
- a row, with focus on the upper mid back and biceps
  - ✓ seated close grip row
- a pull-up, with focus on the upper outer back and biceps
  - ✓ wide grip pull-ups with body weight, or wide grip pull-downs utilizing machine
- a lateral raise, with focus on the shoulders
  - ✓ dumbbells or a lateral raise machine
- a hamstring curl, with focus on the hamstrings and calves
  - ✓ lying hamstring curls either alternate leg or dual leg

You want to do one set of each exercise in sequence (down the list) and then repeat, remembering to keep your heart rate in the 60%–65% range the whole time. If your heart rate drops too low, speed up or jog in place between series.

This workout program may look something like this:

| | Sunday | Monday | Tuesday | Wednesday | Thursday | Friday | Saturday |
|---|---|---|---|---|---|---|---|
| Bench press | | 2 sets of 6 to 8 reps | | | 2 sets of 6 to 8 reps | | |
| Leg presses on a machine | | 2 sets of 6 to 8 reps | | | 2 sets of 6 to 8 reps | | |
| Bent-over rows | | 2 sets of 6 to 8 reps | | | 2 sets of 6 to 8 reps | | |
| Seated wide-grip pull-downs | | 2 sets of 6 to 8 reps | | | 2 sets of 6 to 8 reps | | |
| Machine lateral raise | | 2 sets of 6 to 8 reps | | | 2 sets of 6 to 8 reps | | |
| Lying alternate leg curls on a machine | | 2 sets of 6 to 8 reps | | | 2 sets of 6 to 8 reps | | |

Or something like this:

| | Sunday | Monday | Tuesday | Wednesday | Thursday | Friday | Saturday |
|---|---|---|---|---|---|---|---|
| Incline dumbbell press | | 2 sets of 6 to 8 reps | | | 2 sets of 6 to 8 reps | | |
| Squats | | 2 sets of 6 to 8 reps | | | 2 sets of 6 to 8 reps | | |
| Seated cable rows | | 2 sets of 6 to 8 reps | | | 2 sets of 6 to 8 reps | | |
| Weighted pull-ups | | 2 sets of 6 to 8 reps | | | 2 sets of 6 to 8 reps | | |
| Dumbbell lateral raise | | 2 sets of 6 to 8 reps | | | 2 sets of 6 to 8 reps | | |
| Hamstring curls | | 2 sets of 6 to 8 reps | | | 2 sets of 6 to 8 reps | | |

**Version 1 alternative exercises:**

- an upper body press, with focus on chest, shoulders, and triceps
    - ✓ dumbbell, bar, machine chest press

- ✓ dumbbell, bar, machine incline or decline press
- ✓ machine or weighted dips
- ✓ flat or incline bench dumbbell flies
- ✓ cable crossovers
- a squat movement, with focus on the quadriceps and buttocks
  - ✓ barbell or dumbbell squats
  - ✓ machine leg press
  - ✓ hack squat
  - ✓ Sissy squats
  - ✓ Sumo deadlifts
- a row, with focus on the upper mid-back and biceps
  - ✓ seated close grip machine row
  - ✓ wide grip bent over row
  - ✓ reverse grip bent over row
  - ✓ dumbbell single arm bent over rows
- a pull-up, with focus on the upper outer back and biceps
  - ✓ wide grip pull-ups with body weight (or weighted)
  - ✓ wide grip pull-downs utilizing machine
  - ✓ cable crossover lat rows
- a lateral raise, with focus on the shoulders
  - ✓ dumbbell lateral raises
  - ✓ machine lateral raises
  - ✓ single arm cable lateral raises

- a hamstring curl, with focus on the hamstrings and calves
  - ✓ lying hamstring curls dual leg
  - ✓ lying hamstring curls alternate legs
  - ✓ seated hamstring curls dual or alternate legs

**Version 2**

The home version will utilize exercises you are likely not as familiar with, so if you cannot figure it out, email me.

- an upper body press, with focus on chest, shoulders, and triceps
  - ✓ push-ups
- a squat, with focus on the quadriceps and buttocks
  - ✓ one-legged squats with a chair
  - ✓ squats with an exercise partner or your kid on your back
- a row, with focus on the upper mid-back and biceps
  - ✓ close grip towel rows from a stationary object
- a pull-up, with focus on the upper outer back and biceps
  - ✓ 'jumping' pull-ups (jump up to the bar (chin to bar)) and slowly lower yourself down
- a lateral raise, with focus on the shoulders
  - ✓ lateral or frontal raises (isometric) against a wall
- a body curl, with focus on the hamstrings and calves
  - ✓ body hamstring curls

Do a set of 6 to 8 reps of push-ups, followed immediately by one leg chair squats, then towel rows, then jumping pull-ups, followed immediately by wall resisted lateral raises, and end with body hamstring curls—then repeat that sequence one more time. Occasionally through the series, check your heart rate really quickly to make sure you are maintaining 60%–65% max.

This workout program may look something like this:

| | Sunday | Monday | Tuesday | Wednesday | Thursday | Friday | Saturday |
|---|---|---|---|---|---|---|---|
| Push-ups | | 2 sets of 6 to 8 reps | | | 2 sets of 6 to 8 reps | | |
| One-legged squats on a chair | | 2 sets of 6 to 8 reps | | | 2 sets of 6 to 8 reps | | |
| Towel rows | | 2 sets of 6 to 8 reps | | | 2 sets of 6 to 8 reps | | |
| Jumping pull-ups | | 2 sets of 6 to 8 reps | | | 2 sets of 6 to 8 reps | | |
| Wall-assisted lateral raise | | 2 sets of 6 to 8 reps | | | 2 sets of 6 to 8 reps | | |
| Body hamstring curls | | 2 sets of 6 to 8 reps | | | 2 sets of 6 to 8 reps | | |

## Progression

Once you start to see signs of **RecoverMe**, via how you feel and important follow-up lab work, you can slowly increase your intensity and/or volume to continue to make positive gains and keep the hormones in their optimal state. There are a few ways to do this:

- add an extra day in the week to exercise
- increase the number of repetitions you do per set
- increase the number of sets you do per exercise

Adding an *extra day* in the week might look like this:

|  | Sunday | Monday | Tuesday | Wednesday | Thursday | Friday | Saturday |
|---|---|---|---|---|---|---|---|
| Partner-assisted push-ups |  | 2 sets of 6 to 8 reps |  | 2 sets of 6 to 8 reps |  |  | 2 sets of 6 to 8 reps |
| One-legged squats on a chair |  | 2 sets of 6 to 8 reps |  | 2 sets of 6 to 8 reps |  |  | 2 sets of 6 to 8 reps |
| Partner-assisted towel rows |  | 2 sets of 6 to 8 reps |  | 2 sets of 6 to 8 reps |  |  | 2 sets of 6 to 8 reps |
| Jumping pull-ups |  | 2 sets of 6 to 8 reps |  | 2 sets of 6 to 8 reps |  |  | 2 sets of 6 to 8 reps |
| Wall-assisted lateral raise |  | 2 sets of 6 to 8 reps |  | 2 sets of 6 to 8 reps |  |  | 2 sets of 6 to 8 reps |
| Body hamstring curls |  | 2 sets of 6 to 8 reps |  | 2 sets of 6 to 8 reps |  |  | 2 sets of 6 to 8 reps |

Increasing the *number of repetitions* you do per set would look like this:

|  | Sunday | Monday | Tuesday | Wednesday | Thursday | Friday | Saturday |
|---|---|---|---|---|---|---|---|
| Partner-assisted push-ups |  | 2 sets of 10 to 12 reps |  |  | 2 sets of 10 to 12 reps |  |  |
| One-legged squats on a chair |  | 2 sets of 10 to 12 reps |  |  | 2 sets of 10 to 12 reps |  |  |
| Partner-assisted towel rows |  | 2 sets of 10 to 12 reps |  |  | 2 sets of 10 to 12 reps |  |  |
| Jumping pull-ups |  | 2 sets of 10 to 12 reps |  |  | 2 sets of 10 to 12 reps |  |  |
| Wall-assisted lateral raise |  | 2 sets of 10 to 12 reps |  |  | 2 sets of 10 to 12 reps |  |  |
| Body hamstring curls |  | 2 sets of 10 to 12 reps |  |  | 2 sets of 10 to 12 reps |  |  |

Increasing the *number of sets* you do per exercise would look like this:

|  | Sunday | Monday | Tuesday | Wednesday | Thursday | Friday | Saturday |
|---|---|---|---|---|---|---|---|
| Partner-assisted push-ups | | 3 sets of 6 to 8 reps | | | 3 sets of 6 to 8 reps | | |
| One-legged squats on a chair | | 3 sets of 6 to 8 reps | | | 3 sets of 6 to 8 reps | | |
| Partner-assisted towel rows | | 3 sets of 6 to 8 reps | | | 3 sets of 6 to 8 reps | | |
| Jumping pull-ups | | 3 sets of 6 to 8 reps | | | 3 sets of 6 to 8 reps | | |
| Wall-assisted lateral raise | | 3 sets of 6 to 8 reps | | | 3 sets of 6 to 8 reps | | |
| Body hamstring curls | | 3 sets of 6 to 8 reps | | | 3 sets of 6 to 8 reps | | |

But remember to keep within the confines of the exercise suggestions on time exercising, number of days a week exercising, etc.

## Speed Sets

Speed Sets are another version of MIRTT combining resistance training with cardio with the goal of keeping your heart rate at your personal calculated range. Between each superset, get yourself to a bike/treadmill/elliptical/ etc. and keep your heart rate at the suggested level for 8 minutes. In the example below, I have indicated BIKE as the cardio between resistance training. Do the exercise you prefer. Then return (quickly) to the next exercise/body part and repeat, keeping track of your heart rate the whole time to keep it at the goal. Below is a sample exercise program. Use enough weight on the resistance portion to make yourself work and keep that heart rate where it should be!

As we are in the process of healing, you only need to do this workout plan three days a week, as indicated.

Feel free to change the exercises to fit your gym or what you like to do.

**Day 1**
Bench Press—15 to 20 reps
Triceps Push-downs—25 to 35 reps
BIKE for 8 min
Leg Extensions—15 to 20 reps
Leg Curls—15 to 20 reps
BIKE for 8 min
Cable Crossover—20 to 25 reps
Reverse Triceps Push-downs—25 to 35 reps
BIKE for 8 min
Lunges (wide base) for 45 seconds
Stiff Leg Deadlifts—25 to 35 reps
BIKE for 8 min

**Day 2**
Pull-downs—15 to 25 reps
Standing Curls—25 to 35 reps
BIKE for 8 min
Shoulder Press—15 to 20 reps
Lateral Raises—25 to 35 reps
BIKE for 8 min
Bent-Over Rows—15 to 25 reps
Preacher Curls—25 to 35 reps
BIKE for 8 min
Frontal Raises—20 to 25 reps
Shrugs—25 to 35 reps
BIKE for 8 min

**Day 3**
30 min of Calves and Abs
Long Slow Distance (LSD) for 30 min

## Full-Body CrossFit Program

This exercise program is for those who like to throw their own body weight around. Continue to exercise in the manner of a MIRTT—focus on getting your heart rate to your goal and keeping it there. Do this program two or three times a week. As you recover, increase the number of sets you do of each exercise—that is, go from 2 sets of 20 seconds each to 3 sets of 20 seconds each, etc. For several similar exercise programs to spice up your routine, go to www.drwilley.com and click on *10W* to learn more!

| | Full-Body CrossFit Program |
|---|---|
| Warm Up | 20 seconds of each activity as fast as you can with a 10 second rest between each activity and repeat each one 2 times.<br>• Jumping jacks<br>• Air jump rope<br>• Skipping man (exaggerated)<br>• Knees to chest run in place |
| | 10 second rest |
| Abs | 20 seconds of each activity as fast as you can with a 10 second rest between each activity and repeat each one 2 times.<br>• Reverse crunches<br>• Alternating leg lifts/crunches<br>• Straight leg windshield wiper |
| | 10 second rest |
| Arms | 20 seconds of each activity as fast as you can with a 10 second rest between each activity and repeat each one 2 times.<br>• Cross-chair dips<br>• Chair/table curls<br>• Diamond push-ups on knees<br>• One arm leaning curls (bar, side of wall, towel) (20 seconds each arm) |
| | 10 second rest |
| Core | 20 seconds of each activity as fast as you can with a 10 second rest between each activity and repeat each one 2 times.<br>• Mountain climbers<br>• Crocodile crawl<br>• Push-ups with hip extensions from knees<br>• Jumping jack squats |
| | 10 second rest |
| Cool Down | 20 seconds each set<br>• Standing calf raises<br>• Superman<br>• Squat position calf raises<br>• Wide base upper body twists with arms out<br>• Knee-high march in place |

# Warm Up

Jumping Jacks
Air jump rope – jump your pretend rope

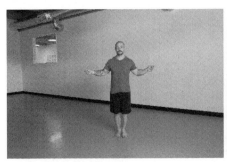 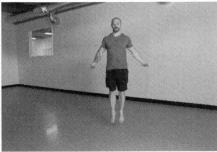

Skipping man (exaggerated) – move around floor

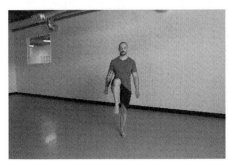 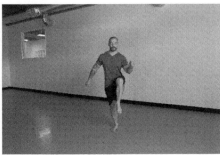

Knees to chest run in place – same as above but run in place

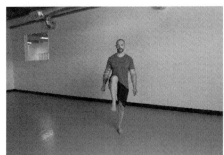 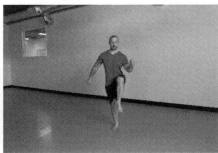

## Abs
Reverse Crunches – start with legs extended and bring to your chest

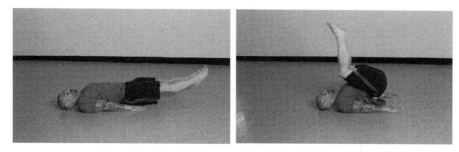

### Alternating leg lifts/crunches

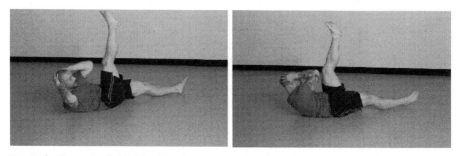

### Straight Leg windshield wiper

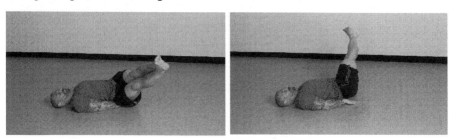

## Arms
Cross-Chair Dips

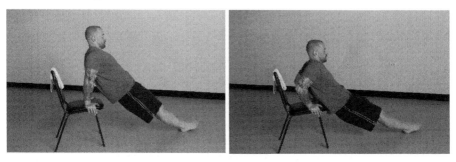

Table/chair Curls – grab a chair, palms up and curl

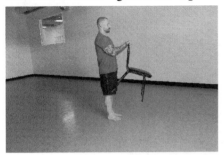

Diamond Push Ups on knees – make hands into diamond shape

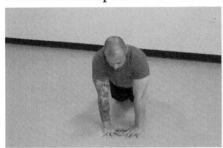 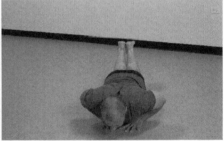

One arm Leaning Curls (Bar, side of wall, towel)

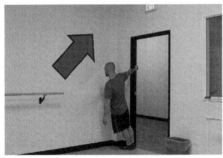 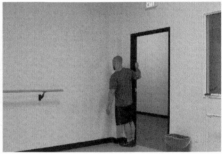

OR (if you are not around a door jamb…)
Isometric Bicep Pose

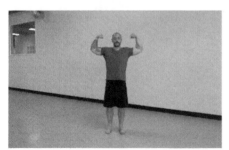

## Core

**Mountain Climbers** – travel across floor as if you were climbing a steep incline

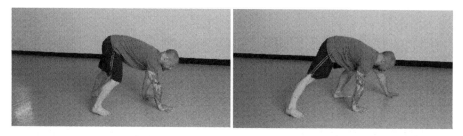

**Crocodile Crawl** – from plank position, feet on towel, travel forward arm-over-arm

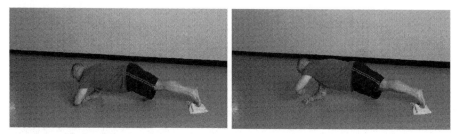

**Pushups with Hip Extensions from knees** – push up position, feet on towel, pull feet under you

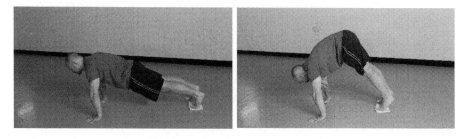

**Jumping Jack Squats** – basic jumping jack with a jump in the middle

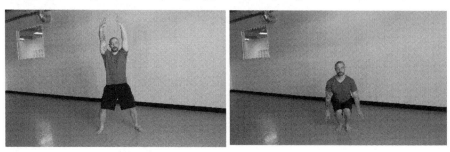

Cool Down
Standing Calf Raises – up on toes, down to heels and repeat

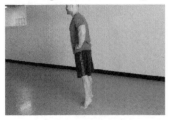

Super Man's – lying on belly, lift legs and arms and hold that position

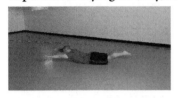

Squat Position calf raises – get in a squat position and up on toes, down to heels and repeat

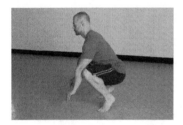

Wide base upper body twists with arms out – hold upper body still and twist lower body

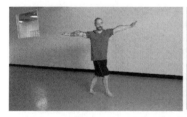 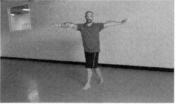

Knee High March in Place

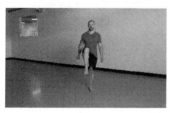

# CHAPTER SUMMARY

In summary, and to repeat what I said at the beginning of the chapter: to recover from your Fat to Fit program, you must start with a good, homemade, stimulant free, pre-workout meal. You must follow the suggestions I made on the post workout meal, as well. Exercise, whatever you decide on doing, must apply these following rules:

- When to exercise
    - ✓ First thing in the morning is ideal, but make it work for your schedule
- Amount of time exercising
    - ✓ Don't exceed 40 min a session
    - ✓ Ideally 20–30 minutes a session
- Number of days a week to exercise
    - ✓ 2 or 3 days a week
- Number of days of rest between exercise
    - ✓ Allow your body to recover for at least one if not two days between exercise sessions
- Multiple training regimens
    - ✓ Change up what you do frequently
- Types of exercise
    - ✓ MIRTT
    - ✓ Resistance training
    - ✓ Cardio or speed your heart rate up training

- Not to exceed 65% max heart rate
  - ✓ Stretching
- Proper exercise monitoring
  - ✓ Keep your heart rate between 60% and 65% max heart rate for the training
  - ✓ Have your doctor run labs to make sure you are recovering

To put it in paragraph form: Exercise when it best fits your schedule (ideally first thing in the morning), two or three days a week, with one or two days of rest between, doing a variety of exercise types, using a combination of resistance training, stretching, and cardio while keeping your heart rate at 60% to 65% max. Don't exceed this, don't under cut this. Period. Trust me—you can increase the amount you do once you have fixed yourself.

There you go—this will start you on your road to recovery using exercise. In the next chapter, I will review the best eating protocols for your **RecoverMe** program following (and during) an over-exercising, undereating program.

# CHAPTER 10
## *RecoverMe* Eating

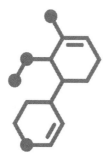

Beyond the obvious, your eating really dictates your overall health. Eat bad, feel bad. Eat too little by counting calories and feel weak and fatigued all the time. Eat the same foods day in and day out, start to develop food intolerances. Recovering from a modern diet and exercise program, or just allowing your body to deal with the daily stressors requires good eating habits. It's not just what you eat. It's not just about what you don't eat. It is what you do around your eating. It's how you eat. It is how you monitor your eating.

There are several excellent eating plans out there that can make you feel, look, and be better. The one I am sharing in this book is one I have had great success with both personally and with clients/patients.

You may be tempted to skip this chapter. We should all know how to eat by now, correct? I mentioned five groups/types of people I wrote this book for because I deal with all five of them almost daily. Let me tell you what each group may be thinking right now, as they struggle to read this chapter:

1. The people who, at one time, trained their backsides off and got into contest/stage shape, did a physique show, a bodybuilding show, or a fitness show and then lost all their effort and cannot get that body back.

Speaking directly to the bodybuilders, physique artists, etc. out there, you are likely thinking, "I can skip this part—I know how to eat. I got into contest shape once, I can do it again. No problem." Well, first of all, there **IS** a problem, as you are reading this book (unless you're reading out of curiosity, or in hopes of helping a friend or loved one). Second, not everything you have read or been taught or seen on the Internet necessarily applies to you. For example: Reverse Dieting. If I had a dollar for every person I have spoken to for whom reverse dieting has failed, I would have a few thousand dollars. Reverse dieting, for those who do not know, is professed by some to be the way out of the low-calorie mess they got themselves into while contest dieting. Just as the name implies, you slowly add calories back into your eating plan under the general recommendation of 5%, or roughly 50 to 100 calories a week. A few inborn errors with reverse dieting: first and foremost, reverse dieting only takes into consideration the calories consumed. It completely ignores the hormonal response to food, the current state of hormonal anguish you are in, the state of oxidative stress your body has just suffered through, the condition of your gut following a pre-contest diet, and the dysfunctional neurotransmitters between your ears. Hopefully, the previous chapters have made you rethink calories alltogether, so you know there is a lot more going on than meets the eye. Not to mention the fact that you just got done with your goal by getting on stage, and now you are going to methodically add 50 calories a week back into your starvation diet? Ain't going to happen. If you are capable of it, I hope you are a lawyer or accountant, as I want to hire you. Anyone who is that anal-retentive and can do that, can count my beans for me.

2. People similar to those above who, no matter what they do, cannot get into bodybuilding, physique, or fitness shape.

The response I classically get from these fine people is, "Well, Doc, I eat very well" (then they proceed to quote, word for word, some diet plan that has some sort of gimmick or limitation I do not care to go into). My question for them is, "Why are you here, then? If you know how to eat, why are you here?" They respond with the classic, "Well, I know it's my hormones or something else diabolical my body is going through, so I want you to figure it out." Of course, I am more than happy to do just that, but inevitably—no—always, we conclude their diet needs to change. Always. The power of the eating plan and its effects (positive or negative) on the hormones cannot be overstated.

3. The ex-college or professional athletes who finished playing their sport, lost all their lean mass and replaced it with fat against their will.

This group of fine people I split 50/50 with their responses. The first half, like the people described above, are pretty set on who they used to be and how it once worked. I call it the Al Bundy personality trait. Living in the past after scoring four touchdowns, etc. I just have to give them a once over with my eyes and they start to listen (in other words, I look them up and down, head to toe with a "really" look on my face, and they get it). The second half knows they have a problem, but blame it completely on themselves for not exercising as much, and letting their diet fail them. As this is certainly involved with their problem, you would now have to agree that is not all there is to it.

4. The people who cannot lose weight, no matter how hard they try, including the good people who used to be thin/lean, but somehow had 20 pounds sneak up on them.

This includes the peri-menopausal/menopausal women, the overworked dads who are doing their best to keep up with their kids, etc. They, like number 2 above, really feel they are eating the best they can, but cannot figure out why they cannot get the poundage off. They are not as slow as group number two at listening to the importance of dietary personalization and modification, but it does take some nudging.

5. The yo-yo dieter whose string finally broke.

These good people are used to changing eating plans every few weeks, so they listen right away. The struggle with them is getting them to stick to the plan for any length of time. I have to convince them to look for other measures of success such as how they feel, body composition, sleep patterns, laboratory findings, etc., rather than the scale or the fact that they don't look like a physique artist in just a few weeks.

So, to answer a question that could be posed in this chapter, "Is this another diet book?"—to that I answer, "No." The **RecoverMe** eating plan following any attempt to get healthy or the body you desire is a dietary solution or cure. It's more than just an eating plan. It is a way of life that really takes into consideration a lot of the fine details that other programs leave out. Consider it a prescription—just like a drug prescription you get from your doctor. Every time your doctor writes you a prescription, he or she knows everything about that drug. The drug's mechanism of action, its potential side effects, interactions, reactions, how long to utilize it, when to take it, what to take it with, etc. That is what this section is about. How to eat to recover.

## General Considerations of a *RecoverMe* Eating Plan

As we have spent the last two hundred plus pages discussing, there are specific criteria your body has fallen into following a Fat to Fit to Fat program. Everyone is a little different—hence the chapter on working this condition up. You need to know how your body responded to your efforts to change your body, and get on the right path to correct the HPA axis adversity, the hormonal havoc, and bowel bollix, as well as reverse the oxidative stress, and clear the toxin trouble.

I cannot write a personalized **RecoverMe** eating plan for those of you reading this book unless you are sitting right in front of me. I have to use these pages to give you the general concepts that I have learned, over the last 25+ years of doing it, that seem to work for the majority of people. I will do my best to give you some pointers throughout to help you fine tune your own program, but consider this the map. You still have to drive to your destination.

The amounts of food I will suggest are *minimum amounts*. Eat some more if you are hungry. ***The RecoverMe plan is NOT restrictive—it is directional.*** My strong suggestion is you get at least what I suggest in, and if you need more, go for it.

Quite honestly when I am asked about calories or amounts of food one should eat, I am a low-calorie, minimal amount guy. I think there is enough good research out there on longevity and health in a lower calorie lifestyle vs. a Standard American Diet (SAD) lifestyle, that more people should pay attention to it. People tend to feel better eating the proper amounts of food vs. what they could eat just because it's there.

We will start with some general suggestions that fall into six categories:

1. What to eat
2. What not to eat
3. When to eat
4. How to eat
5. What to do with or around eating
6. How to monitor your eating

## 1. What to Eat:

There is plenty of room here for smart remarks, so let me phrase it differently for those nonconformists: Eat organic. Eat from this list of foods while you are recovering. Period.

**Animal protein sources**: fresh or water-packed fish, wild game, lamb, duck, organic chicken and turkey, lean organic beef, organic/farm fresh eggs, oysters

**Nuts and seeds**: sesame, pumpkin, and sunflower seeds, walnuts, pecans, almonds, hazelnuts, cashews, nut butters such as almond butter

**Fruits**: whole fruits, unsweetened, frozen, or water-packed

**Vegetables**: all raw, steamed, sautéed, or roasted

**Non-gluten grains and starch**: brown rice, potato flour, millet, quinoa, amaranth, tapioca, buckwheat

**Oils**: cold-pressed olive, flax, safflower, sesame, almond, walnut, pumpkin, coconut

**Drinks**: seltzer or mineral water, filtered or distilled water, herbal teas, almond milk, kombucha

**Sweeteners**: stevia, fruit sweetener, brown rice syrup, agave nectar, blackstrap molasses

**Condiments:** vinegar, salt, pepper, basil, carob, cinnamon, cumin, dill, garlic, ginger, mustard, oregano, parsley, rosemary, tarragon, thyme, turmeric, basically all calorie-free spices

## 2. What Not to Eat (exception: Saturday and Sunday evenings; see below):

Once again, for those mavericks: **DO NOT** eat from this list of foods while you are recovering. Period.

**Don't eat processed food, and that includes**

Anything from a box

Anything in the middle of the grocery store

Anything that has more chemicals in it than a chemist's lab

Anything thatis packaged in plastic, meat included (lunch meat)

Anything that has ingredients you cannot pronounce

**Avoid all refined sugar, high-fructose corn syrup, and evaporated cane juice.**

**Anything that will survive a nuclear war with the cockroaches.**

Basically, anything man-made

**Don't drink alcohol.**

If you do, keep it to fewer than 2 drinks a day, distilled liquor (no beer!). For you weekend bingers, this does not mean you can do 14 on a Saturday night doing some simple multiplication (7 × 2 = 14!).

**Do not drink any form of soda, pop, fruit juice (no matter how healthy the commercial says they are), or energy drink.**

If you drink this stuff for the pharmaceuticals in it (i.e., caffeine), purchase some **Calm Energy** supplements with a large glass of water up to three times a day. (see Chapter 11).

**Avoid all liquid calories.**

**Avoid trans-fats.**

**Do not eat any unwashed fruits or vegetables unless you grow them.**

Pesticides galore out there

**Do not eat soy products.**

Very estrogenic and not good for your thyroid. Your hormones are already messed up.

**Minimize, if not completely avoid, wheat products, including the "healthy" whole grains.**

**If it has been deep-fried, don't eat it.**

**If it was made by a high-school sophomore in a facility with a drive-through, don't eat it.**

**Minimize, if not exclude, all condiments such as salad dressing, ketchup, barbecue sauce, teriyaki, etc. due to all the sugar, gluten, and preservatives they have in them.**

I know what you're thinking. You've heard this before. This sermon is nothing new, yadda, yadda. Your mind is racing with: it's easier said than done, you sound like my personal trainer and my spouse, and now I hate you, etc. Hang in there. These are the gener-alized rules, remember?

The list of dos and don't, as far as food goes on a *RecoverMe* eating plan, can be summed up in one simple sentence:

**If God made it, eat it. If man made it, don't.**

## 3. When to Eat

There is a lot of misinformation out there on when you need to eat: always eat breakfast, never skip lunch, eat 5 to 7 small meals a day, never eat when you are tired—it goes on and on. The truth of the matter is, especially for a *RecoverMe* system following a contemporary diet and exercise program, there are some simple physiological, hormonal, mental, and emotional reasons as to when I suggest you eat.

First and foremost, the overriding rule or umbrella policy of this eating plan is to eat when you can. That's right. Too simple to be true, correct? If I put you on a scheduled eating plan and tell you to follow it, I have just added stress to your life. If you are a type A person, and you miss a meal based on my schedule, not yours, you are likely to have mental and emotional repercussions. A *RecoverMe* program is designed to lower cortisol, not raise it. So, eat when you can. Being an obesity medicine specialist, I can tell you I have just as many successful weight loss clients who eat once a day as those who eat five times a day. It's about scheduling and planning. Plan your eating around *your day*, not my suggestions.

Physiologically and hormonally, there are a few general concepts that work well. If you can do the following, it will help rebalance your circadian rhythm.

- Eat after you fast. Most of us "fast" overnight while sleeping. You break your fast with breakfast. But that does not mean it should be the first thing in the morning, just after you fast. I will be discussing Delayed Eating Techniques or DET below (they are now called Intermittent Fasting after circulating on the Internet).

- Always do a pre- and post-workout meal around exercise. This should be considered as a meal in your day, not supplements or snacks.

- Try not to eat a lot of carbs after 3:00 p.m. unless you are coming out of a fasting period.

- Do your best not to eat within a few hours of going to bed. Going to bed on an empty stomach allows all the anabolic hormones to cut loose and repair your body and brain from the damage caused during the day.

## 4. How to Eat

What? How to eat? I know how to eat there, Doc. Thanks. All joking aside, this is important—we are a fast food society. We wolf down our food, hardly ever chew it completely. In general, we are in a rush, or distracted by the television, cable, the Internet, Netflix, etc. We don't think about *how* we eat. But we need to. You really need to try to turn off all electronics while eating. Seriously. It distracts you and you chew your food about 50% less when your mind is elsewhere. Chewing your food is the first step in the digestive process. Salivary enzymes start their work while you're chewing, and the job of your dysfunctional gut is much easier when it gets chewed up, spit laden food. Do your best not to do anything that distracts you such as driving, working, reading the paper, or the above-mentioned electronics, while you are eating. The one thing I would encourage you to do while eating is to eat with family and/or friends. This adds a unique level of health to your eating that is very hormonally and neurotransmitter friendly.

## 5. What to Do with or around Eating

What to do with or around eating has to do with optimizing gut function, digestion, lowering cholesterol and triglycerides, decreasing postprandial sugar loads and free fatty acid loads to the body (high inflammation, also called postprandial hyperglycemia), and optimizing your hormonal response to your food. It will also help you better your body, obtain/maintain health, lower your heart attack risk, etc. Pretty powerful stuff! This part will include some supplements that I would encourage you to use before, during, and after you eat, all based on your needs and lab results.

**Before you eat:**

Drink 8 ounces of water 20 to 30 min before you sit and eat. Though there is not a lot of scientific data on this practice, anecdotally, it is very helpful. It ensures you get some water in every day. As our bodies have a hard time distinguishing hunger from thirst, drinking a glass of water before eating may slow down your eating and keep the amounts nominal. This is also a good time to remember to add lemon to your water to help optimize your Ph.

You could also consider a cup of green tea for all the health-related benefits. Making it a habit before eating is a great way to get it in every day. Give it a try—I think you will notice a difference.

**Order of food intake:**

The order of your food intake may also be of benefit as you heal from your efforts to get healthy. Although certainly not set in stone, and not a deal breaker with your chances of healing, you may find it does your gut good to eat in this order while recovering:

1. Start each meal with fibrous carbs such as a salad, mixed vegetables, etc. If you are not a big fan, add a fiber supplement such as glucomannan, inulin, or psyllium husk/powder to your meal.

2. After you have consumed about ½ of your fibrous carbs, start eating your proteins and fats (meat portion of the meal) along with the rest of your fibrous carbohydrates.

3. Then (if it is in the eating plan) slowly start your carbohydrates such as quinoa or amaranth.

4. Add jalapenos, habanero, and cayenne peppers to your meal. These all contain capsaicin (gives peppers their "kick"), a chemical shown to help increase metabolism.

**During meals:**

During your meal, plan to take some papaya enzymes, as these will aid in the overall digestive process. As we have discussed, a popular diet and exercise programs destroy the gut. As a result, some survivors have decreased pancreatic function. This little trick really helps the digestive process. If you want to know whether you must do this, do a comprehensive stool test, as I discussed under medical evaluation in Chapter 8.

If you have the bowel bollix we reviewed in Chapter 8, you may benefit from taking oxen bile supplements, especially with large fatty meals, to help the absorption of fat. The test discussed above would also be something to consider if you want to know for sure if you need to take these supplements with meals.

**After your largest meal of the day:**

As I do not want to add to your stress by making you remember supplements with each meal, I will focus on those to use after your largest meal—which for most people is their last meal of the day. Immediately following your eating, at least for your larger meals, you need to have a handful of supplements to help optimize what your body does with the food. PS—this is also what you should do/take any time you eat out at a restaurant or for a Free Window.

When you eat, your blood sugar elevates, as does the level of fatty acids in your blood. This, especially in the presence of foods on my "do not eat" list, can activate adipose (fat) tissue to produce pro-inflammatory adipocytokines, causing inflammation. We are trying to rid ourselves of the high inflammatory state we developed with the overexercising and undereating program, so keeping the postprandial hyperglycemia and fatty acid loads in check will lower inflammation. This is done with gamma and delta tocotrienols at 50–100 mg at your largest meals. I also suggest Berberine at 250 mg with large meals. We will be covering Berberine in more detail later.

Adding Red Yeast Rice in a dose of 1200 mg, along with some Omega-3 fatty acids, with your last meal of the day, will help optimize insulin sensitivity, and increase adiponectin.

Also, soon to be covered in the supplement section is DIM—diindolymethane. We will discuss it in detail in the chapter on supplements in this particular **RecoverMe** program but, as you will learn later, I suggest taking it with your largest meal of the day to optimize postprandial loads and hormonal response to food.

Olive Leaf extract contains many bioactive compounds that act as antioxidants, lower blood pressure, and limit the cholesterol response following a large meal.

After meal supplement suggestions:

- gamma and delta tocotrienols at 50–100 mg
- Olive Leaf Extract 500 mg
- Berberine at 250 mg
- Red Yeast Rice in a dose of 1200 mg
- Omega-3 fatty acids 2–4 grams

- DIM 100 mg

## 6. How to Monitor Your Eating

I am not talking about weighing and measuring your food. I am talking about following your lean and fat mass. To do this, you will need to check the scale, but do not focus on the scale! Measuring and following your lean and fat mass are beyond the scope of this book; however, you can purchase a set of calipers and an instruction booklet on my web site—drwilley.com.

There is another measure of your diet I would like you to consider: Follow your salivary and urine pH levels at least once a week. This will give you an indication if your diet, including your supplements, is adequate in keeping your body and your kidneys in a healthy state so you can function optimally. We touched on pH in Chapter 8, so I will not spend too much time on it here. The pH in your urine should ideally be greater than 6.5 and in your saliva greater than 6.8. If your pH is less than these indicators, you need to increase the amount of vegetables and cut back on meat in your diet. It is a unique, but very cool way to track your dietary intake and supplement intake (minerals), and monitor your overall health.

# The *RecoverMe* Eating Plan

The ***RecoverMe*** Eating Plan is a way of eating for life. It will specifically help someone receeving from a Fat to Fit to Fat program, but it is also something that works for a variety of issues we have touched on. Recall my saying in an earlier chapter that those who survive one of the popular overexercising, undereating programs are like sick people in the hospital. Their blood chemistries, acid/base balance, etc. are all off the charts. So, sick people, people with chronic disease, autoimmune disease, cancers, heart disease, etc. may benefit from this style of eating. I have another book coming out that touches more on each of those specific disease states. It is always good advice to discuss this type of thing with your doctor if you are battling chronic disease, so I am writing this version particularly for the Fat to Fit to Fat crowd.

Not only is this style of eating beneficial for what ails you, not to mention readjusting all the hormones, lowering inflammation, supporting brain neurotransmitters, sex hormones, lowering cortisol, etc.—it is also very easy to do! It allows a lot of freedom. The style of eating allows you to make it work for you and your lifestyle. Imagine! An eating plan that not only works and is specific for your concerns, but that is doable in the long term—something 99% of the diet and exercise programs out there can never claim!

I will start with the style of eating, or how to set up your own eating plan, using the framework I would suggest, and then follow it with some example menus, recipes, and a few powerful case studies to show how others have incorporated these concepts into real life!

The ***RecoverMe*** eating plan has two distinct "tracks." These tracks are designed to help you designate how to incorporate the ***RecoverMe*** eating plan, including frequency of eating, time of day to eat, how often to eat, timing between meals, best body types for the different tracks, other lifestyle things that should be thought of when setting up a lifelong eating plan. These are not set in stone, but provided more as a general guideline for you in setting up your own eating plan.

The different tracks will consist of advice, based on how you assessed yourself and your habits/likes. **Track 1** consists of a more classic breakfast and more frequent meals for you grazers out there. **Track 2** utilizes Delayed Eating Techniques (DET), and is better for those of you who like to or would rather eat most of your food later in the afternoon/evening.

A quick side note on Delayed Eating Techniques or DET: I originally included DET plans in ***Better Than Steroids***, but my editor felt it was better, and easier, to limit the described eating plans to four: The MCD, Isonutroient eating, KETO Runs, and Zig Zag dieting. All good, as this platform is the perfect place for a DET plan!

Although there are a few other rules set in each track, your decision as to what track to follow should be based on the first factor to consider: *What time you eat after waking up, whenever that may be (for you shift workers out there).*

Most Fat to Fit programs participants, fitness stars, and bodybuilders, as well as some other designated health nuts out there, are quite adamant in their belief about meal frequency. Most profess that you must eat at least five times a day for benefit, so let me spend a few sentences explaining why I would disagree, in defense of Track 2:

Genetically we are likely geared for less frequent feedings. Our caveman ancestors most likely were busy hunting and gathering all day, so they could come back to their cave and eat later. Three meals a day was likely invented to manage work schedules of people in factories during the industrial revolution.

There may be some advantages for more frequent meals to your blood sugar if you are diabetic, or for your cholesterol if you have high lipid levels, but there is no research on meal frequency and fat loss or metabolic advantage. The secret to an eating program is it fits your schedule and you can do it. Hence, the two tracks.

For blood sugar issues, I believe it is far better to control your hormones and optimize body comp than it is to worry about eating five times a day. That is the goal of this program. Track 2 may bring up some concerns, as DET could have the potential to burn muscle mass in people doing it. A few studies have shown that less frequent feedings may cause one to lose muscle mass. The most cited one was on boxers. They were in an overexercising, undereating program at the time (exercised way too much and did not recover well), so this program will counteract those concerns.

There is one caution/suggestion I would make. If you decide to follow Track 2, during the middle of your awake fasting time, check your blood sugar. Borrow your diabetic friend's glucometer, go to your doctor's office and have them check it, or go buy one (as I suggested in Chapter 8). If your "fasting" blood sugar is greater than 90 mg/dl, the DET style of eating may not be for you, as it is likely not working to optimize fat loss during your fast. If your "fasting" blood sugar is less than 70, and you feel like garbage, it is also not likely a technique you want to employee in your **RecoverMe** eating plan.

| Factors to Consider | Track 1 | Track 2 |
|---|---|---|
| Eating after a "fast" (usually sleep) | Within an hour of waking or after a workout, after waking—classic breakfast | 8–10 hours after waking up (DET dieting) |
| Meal frequency | 5 to 7 meals, based on your schedule | 2 to 3 meals, based on your schedule |
| Timing between meals once you start to eat | Not greater than three hours | Not greater than 1.5 hours |
| Body type | Lean and more muscular—less fat to keep off | Heavier with a history of difficulty with fat loss |
| Habits | Tends to or likes to graze (eat) all day | Prefers to eat at night, history of skipping breakfast |
| Work Schedule | Regular | Shift work |
| Food based supplements | Per list in Chapter 11 | Per list in Chapter 11, PLUS BCAA 10 grams one or two times during awake fast |
| Medical Concerns | Better for people with diabetes, high cholesterol, etc. | Better for people trying to lose as much fat as possible and still stay healthy |

As I like lists (check lists, to do lists, etc.), I will start with a simple list of things you need to consider while you set up your own ***RecoverMe*** eating plan:

1. Sit down with your calendar and look at your weekly schedule. Chances are, unless you are on vacation or ditching work, your schedule is pretty set all week. You may be involved with different tasks throughout the day, but in the big picture, your schedule is set. What time you get up, what time you go to work or drop the kids off at school, what time you eat, what time you get home at night, what time you go to bed, and when or where your days off fall on the weekly calendar.

2. Map out the five days that have the most similarities in them and are the most consistent for you. Most of us would likely pick Monday–Friday as days that contain the most consistency with our schedules. These are the days you will be following the eating plan most closely. The other two days you will still follow the suggestions, but with a lot more laxity and ease.

3. Do some self-examination—are you someone who likes eating after you wake up—whenever that wake up may be? If yes, you like and want to eat after waking up, you will be following ***Track 1*** of the ***RecoverMe*** eating plan. Track 1 eating plans include menu ideas for what most would classically call breakfast (a.m. eating). If you are someone who does not like to eat right after getting up, you will follow ***Track 2*** in the ***RecoverMe*** eating plan. I have separated these two characteristics out, as food choices will differ, at least classically, and it is very important that you eat to your schedule. One of the biggest reasons people fail to stick to eating plans is the plan dictates their schedule for them, not the other way around as it should be. Both, mind you, are still eating after a fast (breakfast, remember?) which is

what we want, just the time of day differs, so the food choices may differ.

4. How often does your schedule allow you to eat? And how do you feel doing it? If you are someone who can only eat a few times a day, later in the afternoon/evening due to your schedule or how you feel, **Track 2** is for you, even if you like eating in the morning. If you are someone who likes to graze all day so you don't pig out at night when you get home, **Track 1** is for you, even if you don't like getting up from slumber and eating.

5. If you choose Track 2, you basically do not eat for 8 to 10 hours after you wake up. For example: if you wake up at 6:00 a.m.—you will not start your meals until at least 2:00 p.m. If you get hungry or irritable in this time, drink 10 grams of branch chain amino acid (flavored) powder mixed in water.

6. On your schedule, you should now have five consecutive days you are going to follow the *RecoverMe* menu for recovery and repair from your previous diet and exercise program. Decide if you are going to follow Track 1 or Track 2 based on what I just explained.

## General Concepts in the *RecoverMe* Eating Plan:

We need to change some paradigms here with eating—especially for you bodybuilder/physique types and yo-yo dieters. The bodybuilder/physique types call it "cutting and bulking phases" and the yo-yo dieters call it normal. Well, you two groups of fine people, that ain't good for you! Unlike love, where it is better to have loved and lost, than never to have loved at all, it is not better to have lost your fat and then gained it all back again! It is very unhealthy and potentially could lead to several health issues later in life. I have been adamantly opposed to the "cutting and bulking phases" in bodybuilding for years, as they play such havoc on the body and mind. It is not professed by science, but is of the same mentality as the motivational posters on Pinterest and Instagram: no science, just tradition and fluff. Following an intense attempt for ideal physique obtainment, or daily existence for the physique artists, this type of eating must stop. You must develop a lifestyle eating plan, based on scientific facts and acknowledgements, that understands where your body is coming from, as far as all the issues discussed above (hormonal havoc, bowel bullocks, oxidative stress, etc.) are concerned. Would it not be so much nicer to be lean and muscular year-round? Let me add something there: lean, muscular, and healthy! That is what this eating plan helps you do.

In my book **Better Than Steroids**, I outlined an eating plan so powerful, it has helped untold numbers of people not only get the body they want, but enjoy doing so. It is called a Modified Carb Drop of MCD. It is a macronutrient-shifting diet that optimizes hormones, keeps inflammation low, limits gut issues, avoids toxins and the not so good stuff for you, yet still lets you enjoy the occasional "not good for you but tastes so good" food, and to top it off—you feel great doing it. It is a simple plan that calls for a low carb, adequate protein, moderate fat diet for a few consecutive days, followed by a higher carbohydrate, adequate protein, lower fat menu, and repeat. There are many ways to do this eating plan: Two days low carb, followed by one day high carb—a 2:1 MCD—or three days low carb, one day high carb—a 3:1 MCD—or even five days low carb, two days high carb—a 5:2 MCD.

We will *initially* be applying the 5:2 MCD plan to each Track 1 and Track 2. This is why I asked you a page ago to assess your schedule with your calendar. As I said before, my guess is most people out there will choose Monday–Friday as days when their schedule is most set—these will be your low carb, adequate protein, higher fat days, with the daytime both Saturday and Sunday being the same until evening, when we can be a little more lax with higher carbohydrate amounts.

The reason 5:3 MCD works so well for someone coming off a Fat to Fit diet is that their body is in metabolic slow down mode (due to the low calories, certain supplements and drugs), glycogen depleted and extremely insulin sensitive (due to the low carbs a number of modern diet and exercise plans suggest), with high inflammation and hormonal havoc, as we have already discussed. The 5:2 MCD allows for reversal of this perfect storm, in a slow and controlled manner that considers all the metabolic and hormonal disruptions that have occurred (unlike reverse dieting that only focuses on calories).

You are now quite aware that the lifestyle or mother hormones control or override every other hormone out there. As discussed in Chapter 8, leptin, adiponectin, insulin, glucagon, and cortisol all control the hormonal pyramid. The MCD 5:2 plan helps balance and keep these mother hormones in their happy place. For example: the low carb days of the five-day cycle keep insulin and glucagon in a fine balance and the body starts preferentially to utilize fat as its energy source. When insulin is restrained, other things start falling into place such as an increase in testosterone, and lipolysis or fat burning that can take place via glucagon. Adiponectin increases and helps regulate blood sugar and fatty acid oxidation (i.e., you burn more fat!). Leptin starts to balance and allows the regulation of energy, thyroid hormones to rebalance, lowers sympathetic tone, and changes brain activity to lessen the chance of emotional eating and allow more cognitive control of appetite.

The higher fat meals on the five-day cycle of lower carb eating also increase testosterone. Conversely, low fat diets lower testosterone. I have had incredible measured success (checking hormone levels, particularly in men before and after the eating plan was used) with my eating plans described in my book **The T Club** with a diet called The TBT or testosterone boosting therapy.

The higher carb meals allowed on the two days between the low carb days improve the anabolic process by increasing glucose uptake by the muscles, increasing protein synthesis (muscle growth, causing upsurges in the production of growth hormone, testosterone, IGF-1, and serotonin in the brain. It also helps recalibrate leptin which in turn optimizes all the other hormones. Not to mention the fact that it is fun, as you get to enjoy some of your favorite foods (within reason—see below and so on.

The good fat sources listed above as the foods to focus on, are easier for the body to utilize for energy versus the foods with a lot of saturated and trans fats in the opposing list. This means, even though the carbohydrates are lower on the five low carb days, your body will learn to burn a much better fuel source—fat—and you will reap the energy benefits.

Eating in the style or order suggested allows for slower hormonal response to the food and possibly even less absorption of calories. I use an acronym PFF or **Protein, Fat, Fiber** to be included in every meal (except the two days of higher carbs at the last meal of the day—see below). Added to a meal these will slow the insulin response, via a few different mechanisms. In general, all of them will decrease the rate of absorption, thereby slowing insulin's response. Protein also has the additive effect of stimulating the release of glucagon. This antagonizes insulin directly. Fiber can really slow down the rate at which sugar hits the blood stream, thereby causing insulin to respond more slowly as well. If you're not too hip on vegetables, adding a fiber supplement such as glucomannan, inulin, or psyllium husk/powder is a simple way to slow down sugar's hormonal influence. Vegetables add vitamins, minerals, and fiber to your meal and help to change the insulin response. And, like your mom told you, they are good for you!

The *RecoverMe* eating plan following a Fat to Fit program focuses on the good foods that allow the body to decrease inflammation, ensure proper minerals and vitamins like potassium, and provides all the necessary components of a healing program. The list as to how the **RecoverMe** MCD 5:2 eating plan will help you fix yourself goes on and on.

## Putting the RecoverMe 5:2 MCD Together

I should know better than to assume, but I am going to do it anyway: I am guessing most people reading this chose Monday through Friday as their five-day low carb, high fat, adequate protein consecutive days. I have made the sample charts below indicating just that. The tracks will come in later, after you have set your eating plan up as far as what to eat, how much to eat, etc.

Let's first figure out how much we are going to eat. Most of you may automatically think we are going to be discussing calories at this point. Nope. I am most certain that, after reading so far, you know my opinion on calories. They are not nearly as important as they are given credit for. Important, yes—controlling and the end all of eating correctly, no. The last thing your stressed out, cortisol ruined brain needs right now is for you to count calories.

Using the MCD 5:2 eating plan, either with track 1 or 2, you are prohibited from counting calories! I gave you sufficient reasons in Chapter 2, so hopefully you agree. So where do we start designing a **RecoverMe** eating plan following a Fat to Fit program? We will start with some specific generalizations (if that made sense?). I am providing you with the *minimal amounts* of primary/essential nutrients to set up an eating plan. Once you figure this out, you should do your best to prepare at least that amount of food, but allow some leeway for extra if you need it or are still hungry. We do not need to get you back into low amount eating as the crazy diet and exercise program you just did had you do. This **RecoverMe** eating plan allows for free-dom and wiggle room so you feel satisfied and content, not hungry, grouchy, and mad at everything like you while doing or following a Fat to Fit program.

## Monday-Friday or the 5 in the 5:2

I think protein is an easy place to start, but my using the term "adequate protein" likely also got you wondering about the definition. The term adequate protein means the amount of daily protein necessary to meet the needs of the body and keep you in the state of anabolism (growth and repair), but not so much that your body starts turning it to sugar and storing it. I have found this amount to be *approximately* 0.8 grams of protein per pound of scale weight for women, and 1 gram per pound of scale weight for men. Basing protein amounts on lean mass would be ideal, but not everyone has access to body composition.

So a woman weighing 140 pounds would plan to consume *at least* 112 grams of protein a day. A 190-pound woman would need to consume *at least* 152 grams of protein a day. A 190-pound man would consume *at least* 190 grams of protein per day, Monday–Friday. To make that simple to figure out, I have added a chart as Appendix II at the end of the book with protein sources and serving sizes, with amounts listed in grams. **To restate: these are the minimal amounts needed to support the anabolic/recovery process so your body can heal. If you need more, go for it—just be wise in your choices.**

Your primary sources should be:

**Animal protein sources**: fresh or water-packed fish, wild game, lamb, duck, organic chicken and turkey, lean organic beef, organic/farm fresh eggs, oysters

**Nuts and seeds**: sesame, pumpkin, and sunflower seeds, walnuts, pecans, almonds, hazelnuts, cashews, nut butters such as almond butter

You likely noticed that other than in the pre- and post-workout meals, I have not mentioned any protein shakes or protein bars. That is because it is always better to chew your food than drink it in the case of the shake, and bars are processed. If you absolutely must have a protein drink or protein bar because you do not have time to sit quietly and eat your food, as suggested above, here is a brief review of protein supplements so you can pick the correct one for you:

The most common protein supplements available include milk protein (whey and casein), egg protein and soy protein. Whey protein comes primarily as whey isolates, meaning some chemical processing has taken place to "isolate" the protein, making it more available to the body. Whey concentrate, also called intact whey protein, is straight from the nursery rhyme (Little Miss Muffet sat on a tuffet, eating her curds and whey) with a little flavoring added. Whey protein has great bio-availability, is readily absorbed, and causes a rapid hyperinsulimic response. It has an excellent BCAA profile as well as being an excellent source of glutamine. Isolates and Hydrolyates of whey are faster absorbing and, therefore, better for pre-workout, during exercise replacement and post-workout.

Casein is slower absorbing, as are the whey concentrates, and is therefore better for a night time meal, and as a midday meal replacement. It has a slow release effect, as it forms a gel in the gut to slow the transit time of amino acids. Some would argue that this may enhance absorption. Casein also has very high natural glutamine content, and most of the glutamine in casein is found in peptide form for better absorption. Casein protein has been implicated as a problem with autoimmune disease, so if you have an autoimmune condition I would avoid casein. Also, there are many people out there with milk sensitivities, and casein is high on the list of culprits. If you have any concern such as bloating or other stomach issues, get a food sensitivity test, or just avoid casein completely.

Egg protein supplements have a great amino acid profile, but their bio-availability is lower. They are very cheap, which is beneficial; however, they have a very well-known side effect: you are almost guaranteed to lose friends, family, pets, and your job if you use a lot of this protein. Because of its poor bioavailability, intestinal bacteria getting to this has some powerful effects on your fellow man's (or woman's) olfactory system (sense of smell). Need I say more?

Soy protein is not allowed on a **RecoverMe** eating plan as it is very estrogenic and hormonally active. It can also mess with your thyroid, so it is best to avoid it while you are recovering.

All of the protein supplements will advertise vitamins and minerals and additional functional ingredients, but the amounts are of no advantage. Do not include them in your decision to purchase the protein supplement.

Some other important factoids when choosing a protein supplement: avoid baked bars such as bars that contain rolled oats and some granola type bars, as their fat content is elevated and the process of baking denatures some of the protein you are after. Avoid bars with coatings, for example.

In general, the cheaper the protein, the cheaper the protein; that is, you get what you pay for. The whey concentrates are cheaper than the isolated ones and taste a little better because they have carbohydrates and fat in them. Hands down, God-made proteins are the best, such as real eggs, tuna, etc.

For you wonderful vegans out there, this gets a little tough. It is much harder to recover from a Fat to Fit program if you continue just eating carbs. I have a few very successful strict vegans in my practice. They do well overall, as we follow their labs and are constantly adjusting intake based on results and needs. As this becomes very technical and very individual, I chose not to cover it here. Please feel free to email me if you are a vegan and would like more information. Ovo-lacto and lacto vegetarians will do well with this plan.

For fat amounts, we don't care on this plan. Don't worry about them, just make sure you get plenty of them, especially the good ones including the oil sources listed above, nuts and seeds, lots of avocados, egg yolks, fat from your clean, grass fed, hormone and preservative free meats, etc.

For carb amounts, do your best to stay under 35 grams of carbs a day. As it is very difficult to get only 35 grams of carbs in, you may want to consider these carbs the incidental ones that show up without counting them. If you are anal, you could measure out a small amount of carbs from the clean carb list. The important thing here is NO SUGAR!

Some examples of good carbs (above incidental carbs found in some protein sources) would include:

**Fruits**: whole fruits, unsweetened, frozen or water-packed

**Non-gluten grains and starch**: brown rice, potato flour, millet, quinoa, amaranth, tapioca buckwheat

With the fruits, remember to keep within the 35 grams of carbs a day. I know there is a lot of information on carbs in fruit and different effects, after effects, fat effects, etc. In some settings/instances, I agree. In this setting, I have but one thing to say: who cares! Our job is to get you better—we will worry about details later. Eat some fruit everyday—it is good for you!

Eat all the vegetables you can. I said EAT, not drink. A V8 is not a vegetable nor is juicing. Do not worry about the vegetables and their carb amounts.

## Saturday and Sunday or the 2 in the 5:2

This portion of the eating plan makes this really work and more real life. When do most people like to go out and enjoy the finer pleasures of life? The weekends, of course! Unless you are in college, where the drinking starts on Thursday night, this part of the plan works great.

For you Track 1 people, both Saturday and Sunday, from wake up till early evening, should be about the same diet/eating plan as Monday–Friday. Stick with clean fats and adequate protein, but on these days, up until your last meal, do not eat *any* carbs if you can help it.

If you are following Track 2, you have a couple of options here—start your eating earlier in the day, if your schedule allows (i.e., you are not working), as it is the weekend. If you want to keep the DET up on your two-day higher carb days, do your best to get at least one good fat, adequate protein meal in before your carb meal in the evening.

## The Free Window

Sometime in the evening on the two higher carb days you get to have what I like to call a Free Window. From our example so far, that would be Saturday and Sunday.

The free window is an indispensable part of the **RecoverMe** eating program. This can be utilized to your advantage in a few situations, from a dinner party with friends to an important date with your loved one at your favorite restaurant Saturday night.

This portion of the eating plan will allow you to heal from the psychological stress of not getting the body you wanted with all of your effort, as you get to enjoy foods you likely missed or craved while following the restrictive diets. If you are one who generates psychological stress over this type of food, it should be comforting that the free window is a controlled window and, therefore, should not cause duress if you're worried about it. The free window is very powerful physiologically, as well. It will help you repair all your broken hormones following a Fat to Fit program including insulin, growth hormone and IGF-1, testosterone, and your thyroid hormones. It does this in part by helping to increase or balance leptin. It also increases the body's sensitivity to those hormones. In other words, those hormones have a greater effect on the body with the style of eating described.

The lower active carbohydrate intake on the five-day run causes glucagon to increase and thereby burn more fat, while at the same time, causing a decrease and stabilization of insulin, for effi-cient metabolism of carbohydrates and fats. The body responds to this style of eating by increasing the number of enzymes available for essential metabolic processes, including muscle growth and repair, fat burning and utilization and, as some research has shown, an antiaging mechanism by the control of dangerous free radicals. This eating style also acts to detoxify the body by neutralizing, breaking down, and eliminating wastes.

The carb intake during the free window replenishes glycogen stores so you can resume building muscle and getting those growing muscles prepared for the exercise described in the previous chapter.

## How to OPEN the Window

As the *RecoverMe* eating program is about recovery (hence the name) following a Fat to Fit program, you need to begin by opening your window in a controlled and thoughtful manner. I would suggest that, for at least the first three or four weeks after you start the eating plan, and assuming you have done your full medical work up and are on any corrective medications or hormones, and you have read ahead and picked the right supplements for your situation (next chapter), etc., you use the window and have a controlled amount of carbohydrates of your choosing. I would suggest women stick to 100 grams and men stick to 150 grams. Feel free to choose some carbs from the list above—either list—just be sure to keep it controlled for the first three or four weeks. Ideally during this time, you should also do your best to focus on starchy carbs rather than sugary carbs. Having 100 grams of Jelly-Bellies in one sitting is not a good idea. Focus on the starchy carbs such as gluten free grains, brown rice, potato flour, millet, quinoa, amaranth, tapioca, buckwheat, etc. At the same time, do not beat yourself up if you get some sugar in there and treat yourself to a few Bon-Bons.

For these controlled carb binges, do your best to limit protein and fat. We really want the hormonal effect of the carbs at this point. Adding a ton of protein and fat slows things down and can make you feel yucky—think of the way you feel after Thanksgiving dinner, for example.

Whenever possible, avoid combined high fat/high carb meals. I tell my clients "fat is not bad, carbs are not bad—together they are a terror." It is like The Cat in the Hat—the kids were not bad kids, but add The Cat in the Hat with the kids and watch out!

After you have done the 5:2 in the manner described above for three or four weeks, if you are, overall and in the big picture, feeling better, let your window open a little more and start to enjoy more variety for the free window meals on the consecutive two days.

## The *RecoverMe* Eating Plan for a Lifetime?

As you progress in your **RecoverMe** program and start to feel better, start to see improvements in your labs, and your body begins to normalize, you may want to consider changing the MCD day schedule. For example, you are doing great and you want to incorporate another, higher carb day in your week. You could consider adding a higher carb meal mid-week: Start doing an MCD 3:1 or 3:2. If you notice a slowdown in your progress or ability to maintain your goals once you reach them, you may need to consider going back to a 5:2 schedule. I have a few clients who have settled into a lifetime **RecoverMe** eating schedule of 6:1, as it has been the only way for them to maintain their health *and* their goals.

The other way a **RecoverMe** program will work for life is that you will manage all the hormones, gut issues, oxidative stress, and toxins that have been affecting you. You also should learn to give yourself freedom to be real during holidays and vacations. In my book, **What does Your Doctor Look Like Naked?** I covered a chapter on this very topic. As it is one chapter I hear a lot about from people who have read it and benefitted from its advice, I will paraphrase it here.

# Holiday and Vacation Meal Planning and Eating

I get questions all the time about how to eat during vacations and holidays. Clients who are doing very well with their new-found lifestyle and eating habits, are frightened to death to go on vacation, or "make it through" a holiday and blow all their progress.

Let me help relieve you of that fear by pointing out a few facts: the **RecoverMe** program leaves no stone unturned. As you now understand the pathophysiology of the problem, the medical work up, ways to monitor your health and progress with your doctor and on your own, train with your brain, and know how to eat—you also should feel comfortable during holidays and while on vacation.

The MCD 5:2 or, as you progress and change to a 3:1 or some other variation you decide is best for you, is the perfect lead-in to holiday or vacation eating. The consecutive low-carb days prepare your body for the eventual indulgence that occurs during the holidays.

Holidays provide every taste and texture imaginable. I encourage everyone to enjoy all of them. Obviously, that can be a lot of food! So how do we survive holiday eating? Consider a holiday a free window, with one difference: your body needs a little more prep. We need to be sure our "cup" is as empty as possible for a few days leading into the holiday. This is done by following the MCD schedule, as we have discussed above, and using your holiday days as your higher carb days.

First and foremost, holiday and vacation eating should be fun! You are, after all, on vacation, and/or it is a holiday! I have provided some general rules/guidelines below to follow for prepping your body for vacation eating. These rules can be applied to any situation that requires travel or time away from your normal daily activities.

1. REMEMBER YOU ARE ON VACATION!! First rule to remember—have fun, a lifestyle program like this one is just as the words imply: Life, because that's how long it will last,

and style, "a way of doing something." You have the style, now live life!

2. Try to use suggestion number 4 from the ***RecoverMe*** eating plan—***How to eat*** and suggestion number 5—***What to do with or around eating***.

**How to eat:**

Eat slowly. Enjoy your food. Chew it well. Eat with friends and family. Turn off all electronics.

**What to do with or around eating:**
**Before you eat:**

Drink 8 ounces of water or green tea 20 to 30 min before you sit and eat.

**Order of food intake:**

1. Start each meal with fibrous carbs such as a salad, mixed vegetables, etc. If you are not a big fan, add a fiber supplement such as glucomannan, inulin, or psyllium husk to your meal.

2. After you have consumed about ½ of your fibrous carbs, start eating your proteins and fats (meat portion of the meal) along with the rest of your fibrous carbohydrates.

3. Then (if it is in the eating plan) slowly start your carbohydrates such as quinoa or amaranth.

4. Add jalapenos, habanero, and cayenne peppers to your meal. These all contain capsaicin (gives peppers their "kick"), a chemical shown to help increase metabolism.

**During meals:**

During your meal, plan to take some papaya enzymes, as these will aid in the overall digestive process.

**After your largest meal of the day:**

Take the supplements I mentioned above to help optimize the way your body deals with all the "new" foods.

After meal supplement suggestions:

- gamma and delta tocotrienols 50–100 mg
- olive leaf extract 500 mg
- berberine 250 mg
- red yeast rice 1200 mg
- Omega-3 fatty acids 2–4 grams
- DIM 100 mg

1. If you drink alcohol, avoid beer, malt, and ale and only have non-sweetened mixed drinks (i.e., rum in lime water).
2. Continue your exercise program whenever possible!

The *RecoverMe* MCD eating plan, using whatever track works best for you, is really a powerful way not only to recover and heal from the Fat to Fit fiasco, but also to live the rest of your life. It truly is one of those less than 1% eating plans I discussed at the beginning of the book, as it is a real lifestyle and lifelong program and method.

Below I have provided a few sample menus that include schedules for each Track 1 and Track 2 to give you some guidance in doing them. I have used actual clients and included their (brief) stories so you can better relate to them while preparing your menus and *RecoverMe* eating plans.

**Sample menu 1:**

**Track 1, 37-year-old male**

Robert is a pleasant 37-year-old accountant who attempted to get in shape for a physique show. He had a classic case of severe bounce back after doing the show, gaining a whopping 40 pounds within one month of that fateful Saturday, and another 20 pounds the second month following the show. He never took a day off from training because he was worried about the rebound weight gain, as he came from a fat background (he lost a little over 50 pounds in 14 weeks for the show). He felt awful, was having trouble with relationships, and concentrating on his work (he told me he was thankful it was not tax season as, with his current mental state, he would have lost his job at that important time of year).

His labs demonstrated the typical HPA axis disruption and hormonal issues. Subtle insulin resistance and testosterone levels on the far-left side of the bell curve, and a thyroid that was having trouble keeping up. His gut was a mess, and the weight gain was killing him emotionally.

We got things going on the right path with some low dose thyroid replacement, some testosterone boosting supplements, and some calming herbs for his cortisol. I started him on prescription medication for his insulin resistance, fearing that if we did not jump on it immediately, he was going to continue to gain weight.

He cut his exercise back to twice a week with weights and once or twice a week a long walk outside in the sunshine (to boost serotonin).

For the ***RecoverMe*** eating plan following a Fat to Fit diet, he chose Track 1, as he liked a traditional breakfast and his desk job allowed him to eat consistently throughout the day. If he did not plan to eat correctly, he would snack all day on his coworker's M+M's. Track 1 was perfect for him.

This is what his 5 day MCD eating plan looked like (with occasional variations):

| Monday–Friday | Wake up—4 days a week exercise | Menu |
|---|---|---|
| 0630 | Breakfast | Homemade yogurt (made from organic milk) with blackberries and Pea protein |
| 1000 | Snack | Handful of raw almonds |
| 1230 | Lunch | Organic chicken breast with steamed broccoli |
| 1500 | Snack | Pumpkin seeds baked in Cajun spices |
| 1800 | Dinner | Organic wild Salmon with mixed frozen vegetables, salad with oil and vinegar dressing |
| Before Bed | Snack/fiber replacement | Metamucil popsicles |

Saturday and Sunday, or the 2 in the 5:2 MCD schedule, looked like this his first few months:

| Saturday–Sunday | No exercise | Menu |
|---|---|---|
| 0630 | Breakfast | Organic eggs with organic vegetables and elk sausage |
| 1000 | Snack | Mixed berries |
| 1230 | Lunch | Organic Turkey with ¼ cup brown rice mixed in homemade salsa |
| 1500 | Snack | Mixed raw vegetables dipped in organic almond butter |
| 1800 | Dinner—150 grams of carbs! | Amaranth "popcorn" served in almond milk with fruit and honey—a big bowl of it! |
| Before Bed | Snack/fiber replacement | Metamucil popsicles or chocolate pudding |

Over time, and with plenty of medical support for his metabolic derangements (and the occasional appetite suppressant), Robert started to lean-up again. He found that he really could not sway from his eating plan too much, due to his severe insulin resistance. For a few months, he changed himself to a 6:1 MCD to speed things up a little. He wanted to go low/no carb all the time, but I suggested he never do that for longer than two weeks (See KETO run in ***Better Than Steroids***).

Here are a couple of the recipes he used for his eating plan:

**Homemade Yogurt**

> Many recipes on line. Be sure to use an organic whole milk, 2% milk, goat milk, or canned coconut milk. Fresh or raw milk from a reputable source works well too.

**Pumpkin Seeds**

> Simple recipe: Place some raw pumpkin seeds (we stock up on them every Halloween) on a baking sheet after using fat free cooking spray (PAM) on it, single file if possible. Sprinkle Cajun spices over them and bake them in the oven at 350 degrees for about 10–15 min and rotate/flip them over for another few min. Let them cool down and enjoy!

**Amaranth Popcorn**

> Take a medium sized pot with a lid (preferably glass so you can watch things). Warm it up over a stove top on medium heat with just a dash of olive oil (some recipes do not call for any oil, so see what works best for you). Measure out your amaranth grains and add about one tablespoon at a time to the pot. The grains will start popping almost instantly. Move the pot around over the heat so the grains spread out. They should all be done popping in just a matter of seconds. Dump the popped ones out and repeat with the rest until done.

**Metamucil Popsicles**

> Mix two tablespoons of sugar free Metamucil in water.

Oil ice cube tray, using fat free cooking spray (PAM). Fill ice cube tray with mixture to about 2/3 full. Do it quickly or you will have wallpaper paste!

Place tinfoil or plastic wrap over the top and stick toothpicks into the center of each ice cube tray.

Freeze and eat as desired.

## Chocolate Pudding

1 scoop Chocolate protein powder (mixed casein and whey is best)

6 oz. cold water

1 tsp. gelatin

Add Splenda to taste. Blend, place in container in refrigerator for 30 minutes.

## Sample Menu 2:

### Track 2, 42-year-old female

Gina is a wonderful full-time mom, full-time wife, full-time paralegal for a busy law firm, and busy with church activities most days of the week. She was also a self-described yo-yo dieter, who admitted to self-medicating every night after the kids were in bed with lots of sweets—ice cream was her drug of choice.

As her schedule was so busy and she could never get to the gym to do any of the classes she enjoyed, she and her neighbor decided one New Year's to purchase an online, home exercise program (one that has letters and numbers in it). A classic Fat to Fit to Fat program if there ever was one.

In spite of her extremely busy schedule, she managed to get up a few hours earlier to do the exercise program. Her friend suggested doing a no carb type diet while they were doing the exercise program, as she had heard "everyone" loses weight with that type of eating. So, in combination with a low-calorie, no carb diet, strenuous exercise six or seven days a week, and her crazy life schedule, she went for it!

Much to her surprise and delight, she lost weight like crazy for the first few weeks—about 13 pounds. Then it stopped. As is typical, she felt the stall must be her fault, so she cut her calories on her no carb diet back even further and planned to do an extra 30–45 min run after the home DVD exercise program. This meant she got up even earlier than before.

(Do you see where this is going?)

A few more pounds came off, but she could not figure out why she felt swollen all the time. Her stockings were leaving marks on her legs and her wedding ring actually started to hurt, as her fingers were so swollen.

She started to become incredibly irritable with her kids and husband, and even her co-workers wondered what was up, as she was not the same woman she had been. She decided her schedule was too busy, so she stepped down from her church position to get a little more time in the day. Unfortunately, that only made things worse for her mentally, as the guilt was overwhelming.

After a few months of this schedule and being able to avoid self-medicating at night, the ice cream was calling her name. It was the only time she felt good all day long, so that habit started creeping back in. She kept up the exercise out of guilt, but the weight had started to come back, no matter what she did. Finally, her husband told her she needed to come see me. He saw her incredible efforts and it made him sad for his bride. He made the appointment (as she initially refused, and brought her in.

Everything was a mess. She had the incredible timing of starting this crazy overexercising, undereating program; at the same time, she was in a very peri-menopausal state. Her hormones were crazy.

Her gut health stunk. Oxidative stress markers were through the roof—I told her she was a cancer waiting to happen. She was a mess.

We started a detailed and quite extensive hormone replacement regimen, several supportive supplements, and an MCD 5:2 *RecoverMe* eating plan. Exercise was forbidden initially—she had to let her body heal.

With her schedule and habit of eating at night, we decided Track 2 was the best eating plan for her. Here is what her eating plan looked like:

| Monday–Friday | No Exercise | Menu |
|---|---|---|
| 0600 | Wake up—large glass of water with supplements | |
| Noon | 10 grams of BCAA in water | |
| 1500 | Food started | Smoked organic salmon with berries and organic cream cheese (goat) |
| 1630 | Meal #2 | Pea/whey mix protein muffins with almond butter |
| 1800 | Meal #3—Dinner | Organic turkey or chicken, mixed vegetables, a large salad with homemade vinaigrette dressing (easy as her family ate the same thing with her—she only had to make one meal!) |
| Before Bed | Snack/fiber replacement | Metamucil popsicles |

Saturday and Sunday, or the 2 in the 5:2 MCD schedule, had a little more of, what we termed, "family freedom" in it. The family loved to eat out together and part of her healing process was to eat and enjoy her family (and the meals!). She kept up the Track 2 style of eating, as it worked well for her and she felt good doing it:

| Saturday–Sunday | No Exercise | Menu |
|---|---|---|
| 0600 | Wake up—large glass of water with supplements | |
| Noon | 10 grams of BCAA in water | |
| 1500 | Food started | Pea protein shake |
| 1630 | Meal #2 | Homemade yogurt with fruit |
| 1800 | Meal #3—Dinner | Family meal with the in-laws Sundays or out to eat Saturdays. She still tried to monitor total amounts and tried her best to eat in the *style* (order) suggested |
| Before Bed | Snack/fiber replacement | Kombucha |

Over time Gina did well. She certainly felt better and had a much better quality of life. Her weight was very slow to come off, but she was OK with that, as she felt so good and her family was doing well with their mom/wife back!

We added exercise back in at about the 6-week mark, but only a few days a week so we would not stress her schedule too much. As it was early summer, I encouraged all the exercise to be outside with friends and family—not in front of the basement TV.

**Sample Menu 3:**

### Track 1, 36-year-old female

Bethany is a wonderful, full-time school teacher. She began her up-to-date diet and exercise program one summer after school got out, as she wanted to dedicate a lot of time to really getting in shape. Her goal was not for physique purposes. She wanted to become a contender in the Tough Mudder races and similar events. She thought one way to get there would be to start a CrossFit program. She hired a CrossFit trainer and started the paleo eating plan he suggested. Within a few weeks, she became the typical statistic associated with starting a CrossFit program—she was injured. This did not stop her, but it did set her back a little and, as she told me later, it really turned her training up into high gear, as she wanted to make that race by the end of summer.

Bethany put everything she had into it. Since she had the summer off, she literally slept, ate, drank, and trained Tough Mudder! On her rest days, she went for a run, sometimes doing the 10 to 12 miles needed to complete the race. Her diet was the perfect paleo diet, without one ounce of slip up. She and her trainer decided to keep her calories low, so she would be lighter for the race and be able to do a few of the obstacles (her most difficult challenge was anything that required her to pull her own body weight up—like a pull-up).

A few weeks before the race, she had to start getting ready for school and start working on the new curriculum she was to teach that year. She states that was the moment when she knew something was wrong. "I could not focus on the new information. My brain felt foggy."

She completed the race with flying colors, doing very well for her first time and feeling really good about it. Then it happened. She got back to teaching and, although she continued to train hard and eat her perfect paleo, she started to gain weight. She felt fatigued all the time. Her sleep was horrible, as she was consistently waking at 1:00 or 2:00 a.m. and having a heck of a time getting back to sleep. Her school work started to suffer, and when she realized she was not doing the kids any good either, she sought help.

Her OB/GYN suggested she start an antidepressant, convinced that she was just depressed. And although she inquired about her hormones being off, he assured her there was nothing wrong with her hormones. He checked a TSH as she requested a thyroid check, but it was *Within Normal Limits*. He said everything was fine. When she asked why she was gaining so much weight, his response was classic, "You're eating too much!"

She refused to take the antidepressant, as she knew she was not depressed. Other than a normal PAP smear, her doctor did nothing for her.

She eventually came to see me via a friend's referral. We did all the right testing following a Fat to Fit program and she had some issues. She knew that, and felt greatly relieved that the *correct* labs agreed with how she was feeling.

I balanced her hormones, started her on an appropriate training regimen, and had her stop the perfect paleo and start a **RecoverMe** MCD 5:2. She decided on Track 1, as she still enjoyed being active, and she felt she needed a steady supply of food in her to deal with the children. Her schedule allowed her to eat and spend time with the kids, which she really enjoyed. Here is what her initial menus looked like:

| Monday–Friday | Exercise upon awakening—3 days a week | Menu |
| --- | --- | --- |
| 0700 | Breakfast | Homemade yogurt (made from organic milk) with nuts and seeds with whey/casein mix protein powder |
| 0930 | Snack—with the kids | Organic hard-boiled eggs |
| 1145 | Lunch with the kids | Organic chicken breast salad with steamed broccoli |
| 1450 | Snack—school let out | Apple and organic cheese stick |
| 1730-*ish* | Dinner | Game meat (Father and brother are hunters) Mixed vegetables and a large spinach salad with vinaigrette |
| Before Bed | Snack/fiber replacement | Protein muffins |

## Recipes:

### Protein Muffins

1 cup any flavor whey protein powder
3 tsp baking powder
Mix dry ingredients together in mixing bowl.
1 full egg
3/4 c. skim milk
2 T coconut oil
2 T olive oil

Beat the egg, milk, and oils together in a bowl. Make a well in the center of the dry ingredients. Add liquid ingredients to dry ingredients and stir until well blended.

Divide the dough in half (about 3/4 c. dough to each half).

To one half, add 3/4 tsp cinnamon and a heaping 1/4 tsp nutmeg. To the other half, add 1 tsp nutmeg and 1/2 tsp ground ginger. Mix spices into each half until well blended.

Oil mini muffin cups, using organic extra-virgin olive oil non-stick spray. Fill muffin cups with dough to about 2/3 full.

Bake: 425 degrees for 6 minutes

1 muffin from a 12-dish muffin pan: 85 calories

5 g fat

2 g carbs

8 g protein

31 mg sodium

## Sample Menu 4:

### Track 2, 49-year-old male

Shawn is a very active security/police officer who, like most shift workers, started feeling the effects of his crazy schedule a few years into his career. He floated between day shifts, swing shifts, and night shifts, based on scheduling, time of year, and other officers' vacations.

He had always exercised and trained hard, since high school, but he felt as if things were changing on him. His body was not responding like it used to, his strength was down, his moods were erratic, and he just did not feel well overall. So, he went to his doctor.

His primary care doctor diagnosed high blood pressure and high cholesterol and told him that was why he was feeling so terrible. He was started on a statin and a blood pressure medication. Needless to say, this just made him feel worse.

His buddies convinced him it was due to "Low T" as they all had found the fountain of youth in testosterone replacement therapy (TRT). He found a clinic online that does nothing but replace men's testosterone, and went in for a visit. He was convinced by the nurse practitioner (NP) who saw him that all his symptoms were due to his testosterone, and even though his levels were normal (total testosterone was 475 ng/dl), they were too low and he needed them higher. He started taking the shots as prescribed.

Initially, it was the fountain of youth! He felt great! Strength came back, energy was good, his moods improved. Over time, however, he felt the shots were not working as they once had. The NP increased his amounts, but this just made him gain a lot of weight and become grouchy (in his words). It also made his blood count sky rocket. A condition called erythrocytosis.

He started feeling that terrible fatigue again, to the point his primary care doctor prescribed him Adderall (legal speed/methamphetamine), to help him stay awake at work. It did help him for a few hours after taking it, but then he started crashing mid awake cycle and then, paradoxically, it made it impossible to sleep. So, in typical western medicine form, he was prescribed a sleep aid (for every drug side effect, there is another drug).

He felt terrible. He literally felt as if he were dying and could not keep going at this rate. He finally found his way to my office and, after a few months waiting time to get into see me, we met.

Keeping the story short—I got him off all the drugs, started him on some supplements to help balance his hormones out, started something to re-energize his testosterone production, got him on a controlled exercise pattern, and we started a **RecoverMe** eating plan, Track 2, as it worked best with his alternating shift work.

We made the low carb/high carb days work this way to fit his schedule: On days he worked, no matter what the time, he would always wake up and fast for 8 hours, using a DET schedule, but have a large glass of water with 10 grams of BCAA in it every two-three hours. He would then fit his meals in during the last part of his "day" (about 6 hours) before going back to bed (again, whatever time that may have been).

| Work days/nights | Moderate Exercise | Menu |
|---|---|---|
| Time varied | Wake up—large glass of water with supplements | |
| Time varied (but every 2–3 hours) | 10 grams of BCAA in water | |
| 6 hours before going to "bed" | Food started (he loved traditional breakfast food, no matter what time of day) | Organic eggs with organic turkey bacon, protein muffins with almond butter and sugar-free jam |
| 1–2 hours later | Meal #2 | Casein/whey mix protein drink with berries and a handful of nuts |
| 1–2 hours later | Meal #3 | Organic turkey, chicken, or beef with mixed vegetables and a large salad |
| Before Bed | Snack/fiber replacement | Protein drink with psyllium powder in water |

His days off from work would be his higher carb days. He would occasionally use Track 1 style of eating, but he found Track 2 style of eating using the DET as something he liked and it did his body good, by his report.

He really did not follow any menus on these days, as it just worked better for him. He ate good, clean, starchy carbs in the evening, and limited fats and proteins with them. He loved the pump this gave him in the gym the next morning, so he kept it up.

His hormones came back to normal, his strength returned and, although he is no longer 25, he feels great—even with the shift work. PS—he is on no prescription drugs or medication.

# SUMMARY

After your body suffers through any of the overexercising, undereating suggestions out there, or any severe stressor for that matter, you must allow healing time. It does not happen overnight. It really is a big picture thing, with everything we have discussed so far and including what we are going to discuss next—the suggested supplements, sleep, and putting it all together. But the diet should lead the charge in your recovery. I would suggest starting the eating plan even before the workup is done with your doctor (or a doctor), as part of the hormonal balance, fixing the gut, limiting oxidative stress, etc. starts with a good eating plan.

Remember what the father of modern medicine, Hippocrates said:

*Let food be your medicine, and medicine be your food.*

# CHAPTER 11
## *RecoverMe* Suggested Supplements

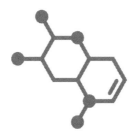

I use a lot of different nutritional and herbal supplements in my practice. I think they allow an integration of medical practices from around the world, and really do a lot to help people get and stay healthy. I must admit, however, that for a long time I was a food purist. I would suggest you just eat really well and you would not have to take any supplements. As this is all but impossible now-a-days, supplements have a wonderful role in attaining and maintaining health.

There are literally *thousands* of supplements I could cover, as I use supplements in my practice for every condition I run into, but my focus will be on those that I have found help in the ***RecoverMe*** package following a Fat to Fit to Fat program.

My suggested supplements for anyone after a very valid attempt to get in shape is based on the fact that most people who come to me in this manner of a train wreck, have many of the same issues and deficiencies. Therefore, it is likely beneficial to suggest these supple-ments to everyone following a bout of overexercising and undereating. In doing this, I am making a few assumptions. I am assuming you are insulin-resistant for example, as most people in this situ-ation are, even if they don't fit the phenotype (look like it), or the standard labs say you are not. That is why I suggest more advanced testing, such as checking adiponectin or a toxicology screen. If you have regained a lot of weight in a short time after your Fat to Fit to Fat program, chances are you are insulin resistant.

Obviously, as I discussed in detail in Chapter 8, it's best if you do the nutrient, bowel, and hormone testing before starting the supplements, as that will allow you and your health care provider to really hone in on what you need personally. For example: you will notice the first supplement I suggest for everyone is magnesium. The dose and form I am suggesting is very rudimentary, as I know you need it, but the only way to find out how much you need is via the RBC Mg+ test I talk about in Chapter 8. The form it comes in is also variable. I will suggest a glycinate form, as it tends to give fewer bowel issues (compared to magnesium citrate or magnesium oxide), but you may be better off with magnesium threonate, based on your situation. Make sense? It really is the absolute best option to get things checked first, so you can personalize your treatment! I highly recommend it!

I am often asked, "Should I continue with the supplements I am already on?" That is a very good question. If I could see your list, I could tell you more specifically; however, as that is impossible in this setting, I would recommend you continue them until you have a chance to discuss it with a professional in your area. There is likely some crossover with those I am going to suggest and those you are taking, so you may have to do a little research on your own.

It can add up to several pills that require swallowing a few times a day. That is not pleasant to everyone, due to a great gag reflex, transportation problems, resulting reflux and "powder burps" following, etc. So, I have a few suggestions: if the load is too big, spread them out. If you really hate swallowing pills, see if you can find the sug-gested supplement in powder form. Most, if not all, supplements can be found in powder form (the exceptions being the fat-soluble vita-mins and Omega-3 fatty acids), and it's easy to put them into your drink and down them that way. I claim no responsibility as to how it will taste. There are companies out there that will do this for you. Make a list of your supplements, and either through your doctor or their online web site, you can have all of them made into powder form for drinking, or any other delivery method that makes more sense for you and your situation.

You may notice that a few of the supplements I discussed in the book are not on this list. For example: prebiotics and probiotics. As I described earlier, these can be (and should be) a very personal thing. You really should be tested to see which ones you need and then plan to rotate them on a regular basis. I also mentioned that I think the best way to get good probiotics in your system is to make them with homemade yogurt, kombucha, etc. Some of the other supplements I have listed earlier in the book can/should be used for specific situa-tions, and therefore will not be on this list below.

I will provide a chart with the supplements listed in the catego-ries above, then get into more detail on each supplement following. I will do it in this order:

1. Supplements that should be considered for everyone following or after a Fat to Fit program

    a. I will indicate those which may be more applicable to you by starring them (*) to give a little more specificity in your decision to take them or not

    b. The ones not marked with an (*) should be considered by everyone

2. Specific supplements for men and women of different ages

*Before taking any supplement, it is imperative that you visit with your doctor to review them and how they pertain to your specific health and situation! This is a must! Several of these supplements in my list are prescription drugs in other parts of the world and have many drug-to-drug, drug-to-supplement interactions so be wise! Please seek professional advice before taking any of them.*

*RecoverMe* Supplements following a Fat to Fit program:

| Supplement | Dose | Time of day to take it | How long to take it | What it does |
|---|---|---|---|---|
| Magnesium Glycinate | 400 mg | Once a day | Forever if you continue exercising | Replaces valuable minerals and keeps pH up |
| Vitamin C | 1000 mg | Twice a day | Forever | Antioxidant |
| Calm Energy | 1 pill | Twice to three times a day as needed | As needed for clean, calm energy | Natural source of caffeine and calming herbs to minimalize potential caffeine side effects |
| B-Complex | Varies | Twice a day | Forever | Important vitamin in many metabolic actions in the body |
| Multivitamin with minerals | Varies | Once a day | Forever | Replenish nutrients |
| N-AcetylCystine (NAC) (take with your vitamin C) | 600 mg | Twice a day | Three to six months | Heals the liver, rate limiting step for the formation of glutathione (strong antioxidant) |
| L—Glutamine | 5000 mg | Three times a day | Forever, if you continue to exercise or have gut issues | A lot. See below |
| *Boswellia (standardized to 65% boswellic acid) | Up to 900 mg | In divided doses, twice a day | At least three months | Anti-inflammatory for whole body, including gut |
| **Relora | 250 mg | Three times a day | At least three months | Lowers cortisol |

| **L-Taurine (Amino Acid) | 3000 mg | Once or twice a day | At least three months | Used for replacement and keeps the sympathetic nervous system toned down |
| ***Acetyl-L-Carnitine | 1000–3000 mg | Twice a day | Three to six months | Supports mitochondrial function |
| ****Berberine | 250 mg | Two to three times a day | Three to six months | Helps with insulin resistance and acts as a strong anti-inflammatory |

\* Use if you are achy and sore, have joint pain, or bowel issues
\*\*Use if you are under high stress, anxious, wake every night between 1:00 and 3:00 a.m.
\*\*\*Use if energy is a big issue or you are severely fatigued all the time
\*\*\*\*Use if you have been diagnosed with insulin resistance and/or cannot lose fat

## Magnesium Glycinate

Magnesium is involved in over three hundred different metabolic processes in our bodies including, but not limited to: ATP production, oxygen uptake, central nervous system function, electrolyte balance, glucose metabolism, muscle function, heart rate and function, and bone density.

Our diet tends to be lacking in it and following a concentrated diet and exercise program (or any athletic endeavor), it is low—sometimes very low, which is why you need to get it checked via a RBC Mg+ level.

## Vitamin C

There is so much research on vitamin C, I do not know where to begin. Fact is—you need more than is required to prevent scurvy, as the fine government recommends, especially to recover and start feeling better. You should also take it with your NAC (see below), so you don't get cysteine kidney stones. Those are not fun.

## Calm Energy

Calm Energy is a unique combination of natural caffeine and calming herbs such as L-Theanine and passionflower extract. It was designed to increase energy, wean oneself off energy drinks and/or pop, without the side effects commonly associated with caffeine, such as a rapid heart rate, nervousness and jitters, etc. As your efforts to get healthy or the body you want really puts the energy in the toilet, this is a great supplement to help you function while you are recovering.

## Multivitamin with minerals

This is just a good idea in general, with our current food status, and even the western medicine gurus suggest a multivitamin a day. Make sure yours has minerals in it to help keep your pH where it should be.

## Boswellia

This is one of my favorite supplements. The resin, obtained from tapping the Boswellia tree (native to north Africa and the middle east), is called Frankincense. As you likely recall from the Good Book, this was one of the gifts the Three Kings gave to baby Jesus (so you know it is good stuff!). It acts as a powerful anti-inflammatory for your joints, muscles, and gut. It is an absolutely essential product following a Fat to Fit program.

## Relora

Relora is a combination of philodendron and magnolia—two traditional Chinese herbal remedies. Relora has been shown in blinded, controlled studies, to decrease cortisol and help the body manage the stress response. As your body is in a cortisol bath following (and during) an overexercising, undereating program, this supplement is a must to help you recover.

## N-AcetylCystine (NAC)

NAC provides the body/liver with the amino acid cystine. Cystine is the rate limiting step (meaning the reaction cannot take place without it) in the formation/production of glutathione. Glutathione is arguably the strongest, most important antioxidant in the body. As you are in a very deep state of oxidative stress, with your popular diet and exercise program, this supplement is a must.

## Acetyl-L-Carnitine

L-Carnitine is an amino acid that transports fatty acids to the mitochondria for processing into energy. It is also used for a variety of other medical conditions such as heart disease. Your body can make it as needed, but in certain medical conditions, and in a person recovering from a Fat to Fit program, this amino acid becomes essential, as the body in this state cannot make enough of it. It also acts as a strong antioxidant to help counter the oxidative stress of overexercising and undereating.

## Berberine

Berberine is an alkaloid extracted from plants and has been used in traditional Chinese medicine for years. It has strong anti-inflammatory properties, and helps reduce glucose production in the liver (similar to the drug metformin). It can also help to lower cholesterol. It is a great adjunct, as I mentioned in Chapter 10, to use after your largest meal of the day, especially if it is a free window or cheat meal, as it helps balance the post prandial eating effects on the body.

## L-Taurine

This is another "non-essential" amino acid that becomes essential to you following a Fat to Fit program. Taurine acts as an inhibitory neurotransmitter and helps tone down the sympathetic nervous system. It supports the insulin receptors and benefits glucose metabolism, increases antioxidant response, helps balance the inhibitor neurotransmitter GABA, and acts as a natural diuretic.

## L-Glutamine

This is yet another "non-essential" amino acid that becomes essential to you following vigorous diet and exercise. L-glutamine optimizes metabolism, repairs and helps heal tissue, maintains muscle mass, is needed to make DNA, supports the immune system, is needed for a healthy gut, is important for acid-base balance, is a precursor for GABA (primary relaxing hormone in the brain), and the list goes on!

This amino acid is an absolute must for you to fully repair and heal. It's best taken on an empty stomach, in powder form, in a large glass of water.

## Supplements for Specific Groups of People

As we get wiser (I don't like "get older"), our bodies change. Hormones change or go away completely, and that changes the needs of the body. Toxins have more time to build up, as do the effects of oxidative stress (that wrinkled skin come out of nowhere? Did you wake up with grey hair?).

Once again, writing to the masses on specific recommendations is tough business! I have found in the past, that separating it into sex and age groups, less than 40 years of age, greater than 40 years of age, seems to work well—so—that is what I will do right now!

A lot of the supplements are listed in both sexes and age groups, but be sure to pay attention to dosing, as this is where it differs a little.

## Males Less than 40 years of age

| Supplement | Dose | Time of day to take it | How long to take it | What it does |
|---|---|---|---|---|
| DIM | 200 mg | Once a day with largest meal | Three to six months | Balances hormones, particularly estrogen metabolism |
| Cordyceps sinensis | 2000–3000 | Twice a day | Three to six months | Improves immune function, improves stamina and athletic performance, improves liver function |
| Eurycoma longifolia | 200 mg | Twice a day | Three to six months | Antiestrogen effects, possible testosterone booster |
| Melatonin | 5–10 grams | At night before bed | Three to six months | Strong antioxidant and sleep aid |

## Males greater than 40 years of age

| Supplement | Dose | Time of day to take it | How long to take it | What it does |
|---|---|---|---|---|
| DIM | 300 mg | Once a day with largest meal | Three to six months | Balances hormones, particularly estrogen metabolism |
| Cordyceps sinensis | 2000–3000 | Twice a day | Three to six months | Improves immune function, improves stamina and athletic performance, improves liver function |
| Eurycoma longifolia | 400 mg | Twice a day | Three to six months | Antiestrogen effects, possible testosterone booster |
| Alpha lipoic Acid (ALA) | 200–400 mg | Twice a day | Three to six months | Strong antioxidant, balances sugars |
| Melatonin | 5–10 grams | At night before bed | Three to six months | Strong antioxidant and sleep aid |
| Omega-3 fatty acids | 5–10 grams | In divided doses throughout the day | Three to six months | Membrane integrity, heart health, brain health |
| Phosphatidylserine | 300 mg | At night before bed | Three to six months | Improves brain chemistry, fights depression |

## Females less than 40 years of age

| Supplement | Dose | Time of day to take it | How long to take it | What it does |
|---|---|---|---|---|
| DIM | 100 mg | Once a day with largest meal | Three to six months | Balances hormones, particularly estrogen metabolism |
| Cordyceps sinensis | 1000 mg | Twice a day | Three to six months | Improves immune function, improves stamina and athletic performance, improves liver function |
| L-Tyrosine | 1000 mg | Two to three times a day | Three to six months | Helps control cravings/appetite |
| Melatonin | 5–10 grams | At night before bed | Three to six months | Strong antioxidant and sleep aid |
| L-Theanine | 200–400 mg | Three to four times a day | As long as needed | Calming/anxiety-reducing agent |

## Females Greater than 40 years of age

| Supplement | Dose | Time of day to take it | How long to take it | What it does |
|---|---|---|---|---|
| DIM | 200 mg | Once a day with largest meal | Three to six months | Balances hormones, particularly estrogen metabolism |
| Vitamin D3 | 2000 IU | Once a day | Lifetime | Bone protection, hormone modulator, lots of other stuff |
| MK-7 | 90 mcg | Once a day | Lifetime if needed | Active vitamin K—supports bones, heart health, etc. |
| Cordyceps sinensis | 1000 mg | Twice a day | Three to six months | Improves immune function, improves stamina and athletic performance, improves liver function |
| L-Tyrosine | 1000 mg | Two to three times a day | Three to six months | Helps control cravings/appetite |
| Melatonin | 5–10 grams | At night before bed | Three to six months | Strong antioxidant and sleep aid |
| L-Theanine | 200–400 mg | Three to four times a day | As long as needed | Calming/anxiety-reducing agent |
| Phosphatidylserine | 300 mg | At night before bed | Three to six months | Brain enhancer, helps with depression |

## *Cordyceps sinensis*

Cordyceps is a medicinal fungus or mushroom. Not to make you ill, but it is grown on the backs of caterpillars. It is a strong antioxidant, helps increase energy levels, improves stamina and endurance, and can treat/benefit muscle aches and soreness. It can also claim being of benefit to the immune system and helping detox the liver. It is the perfect supplement following a Fat to Fit program, and possibly for life in some people.

## *Eurycoma longifolia*

Eurycoma (also known as Tongkat Ali) has antiestrogen effects and may be effective in helping erectile function (especially after AAS use). There are claims of it working as a testosterone booster, but it is hard to find studies on this effect. Anecdotally, I have had many men's T levels come back much higher after using this supplement, but they were undertaking the entire program, which definitely increases T levels. As libido and erectile function are not optimum if you destroyed your testosterone either by taking AAS or just have to high of cortisol with all the low calorie dieting and aggressive exercise this supplement fits in nicely.

## Phosphatidylserine

Phosphatidylserine contains amino acids and fatty acids. It helps build and protect cell membranes and is of particular importance in the brain. It has been shown to slow the rate of cognitive decline, battle depression, and may even improve athletic performance. I have had great luck in practice with it in men and women stressed to the hilt and having a hard time sleeping due to the ADD (Attention Deficit Disorder) that tends to affect them at night.

## DIM

Cauliflower, cabbage, broccoli, bok choy, brussel sprouts, green leafy vegetables (and other members of the Brassica family) all contain a chemical called diindolymethane or DIM. DIM promotes beneficial estrogen metabolism in men and women by reducing the levels of 16OHE1 and 4OHE1—bad estrogens—and increasing the formation of 2OHE1—the good estrogen. As hormone metabolism is so messed up with a Fat to Fit program, this supplement really helps get things balanced over time. DIM is also beneficial, as it frees up more available testosterone by reportedly displacing testosterone from SHBG, thereby making more free T.

## MK-7

This is vitamin K2, known as menaquinone, the more active form of vitamin K. It has a much longer half-life than K1 (days vs. hours), is better absorbed than vitamin K from green leafy vegetables, and is supposedly more active than regular vitamin K. I am suggesting this for females greater than 40 years of age, as the high stress and meager hormones that occur with any attempt for body perfection can be very detrimental to bone health—I see a lot of osteopenia and osteoporosis in these good people. Younger women and men are also at risk, but this is the age group I have seen it in the most.

## Vitamin D3

Everyone is familiar with Vitamin D3. It is the active form of vitamin D—the same one your body makes when you are exposed to sunlight. Nothing beats sunlight for increasing vitamin D (and for so many other reasons—one of the reasons why the exercise prescription in Chapter 9 encouraged outside exercise activity whenever possible). Vitamin D is usually low in Fat to Fit survivors just due to general health reasons. As it acts more like a prehormone in so many aspects of your well-being, it suffices to say here—you need it. Get levels checked for optimal dosing.

## L-Tyrosine

L-Tyrosine is a non-essential amino acid the body makes from another amino acid called phenylalanine. L-Tyrosine is an essential component in producing neurotransmitters including epinephrine, norepinephrine, and dopamine—all depleted in an overexercising, undereating program. It has been shown to help replenish these hor-mones in/after a high-stress situation. It seems to help with cravings and hunger as well. The reason a lot of people self-medicate with Bon-Bons at night is to raise these very neurotransmitters. L-Tyrosine also helps with overall hormone balance, including adrenal hormones, thyroid hormones, and pituitary hormones.

## Melatonin

Melatonin is produced in a little gland at the end of your optic nerves in the back of your head called the pineal gland. It is a very strong antioxidant, hence its use in this situation, as well as a sleep aid. Melatonin helps regulate your circadian rhythm—when it gets dark, the pineal gland secretes melatonin to help you sleep—hence the reason it is a good idea to go to bed when the sun goes down and stop all screen time—especially cell phones, iPads, computers, etc. when it's dark outside, as these all have blue light that fools the pineal gland into thinking it is still the middle of the day.

## Alpha Lipoic Acid (ALA)

ALA is an essential fatty acid found inside every cell in the body. It is needed to produce energy, optimizes blood sugars and carbohydrate metabolism, and is a powerful antioxidant. Animal studies show it may be of benefit for optimal thyroid function. It also allows other antioxidants to "recycle," in particular, vitamin E, vitamin C, and glutathione. I have suggested it in males over 40, as this group of people, anecdotally, seems to benefit from it rather well.

## Omega-3 Fatty Acids

The best source of Omega-3 fatty acids is cold water fish, but as it is hard to eat enough organic fish, supplementing Omega-3 fatty acids works well. Omega-3 fatty acids reduce inflammation and are very important for brain function. Low levels of Omega-3 fatty acids show up as symptoms such as fatigue and mood swings, poor mem-ory, dry skin, etc. Sound familiar following that Fat to Fit program? Dosing is high for optimal levels and taking that many fish oil pills a day could ruin your kissy-face relationship (you stink when you burp), so freeze the pills and spread them out throughout the day. Get your Omega-3 Index checked by your doctor for optimal dosing and maintenance.

# SUMMARY

In summary, we have covered a lot of supplements here. We could have, and possibly should have, covered more. The classic scenario will occur the day after or possibly the same day I release this book: "Doc Willey—you did not mention supplement XX and that is what you put me on to help me lose my fat after my yo-yo dieting! Why didn't you mention it?" Unfortunately, I cannot mention every supplement out there. There are too many, or some are controversial, or some have too many drug interactions, etc. These supplements I have revealed are, overall, safe and effective. But even these—every one of them—needs to be cleared by your doctor before you take them! I cannot emphasize that enough.

I also did not want this to become a supplement review book, so I kept the lists to the most effective and safe ones.

My last supplement suggestion is this, take a supplement holiday every once in a while. I think supplement holidays are a really good idea. They help prevent the monotony of taking supplements day in and day out, they allow for some cost savings, as supplements can get expensive over time, and they give your body a break so you don't get used to the supplements—a condition called tachyphylaxis—it is when your body becomes accustomed to a supplement or drug, and the supplement or drug stops working. Alcohol is a great example. The first beer an alcoholic ever drank gave him or her a nice buzz. Over time, to achieve that same feeling, he needs to drink two quarts of Vodka. That is tachyphylaxis.

In the final chapter of this book I will summarize putting the whole **RecoverMe** plan together, I will mention when to wean yourself off certain supplements but, as a rule, I would suggest you adopt one of the following supplement holiday schedules:

1. Take every Sunday off from your supplements
2. Take a week off every month or two from your supplements

As I said above, I think you will notice a difference, both in their effectiveness and your wallet, by taking the occasional supplement holiday.

One last time as I must emphasize it again:

*Before taking any supplement, it is imperative that you visit with your doctor to review them as they pertain to your specific health and situation! This is a must! Several of the supplements on my list are prescription drugs in other parts of the world and have many drug-to-drug, drug-to-supplement interactions, so be wise! Please seek professional advice before taking any of them.*

# CHAPTER 12

## *RecoverMe* Sleep

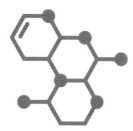

If you want to recover from your high-stress life that you just made worse by inappropriately trying to exercise more and eat less to get the body you want, you need sleep. If you want to change your body, lose weight, get stronger—you need to sleep. If you want to feel good, have stable emotions, and contribute to others in life—you need to sleep. Sleep is so important, this could easily have been the longest chapter in this book. I cannot emphasize enough the importance of a good night's sleep.

**I am going to mention several supplements and even some drugs that will hopefully better your sleep experience. The lists I have provided are for you to pick and choose from—*not take them all at once!* Use the lists as a resource to find what works best for you. You also need to review your chosen sleep aids with your doctor. This is of extreme importance!**

Sleep does several things, including enabling the anabolic process, restocking neurotransmitters, regulating the immune system and function, removing toxins and byproducts of metabolism, and allowing the brain to process all the information it receives during the day.

Studies have shown that up to 700 genes change when your sleep is poor. This is important, as your quality and time spent sleeping can influence your genetic expression. I briefly review other things that change your genes in Chapter 13 in the FAQ section.

Almost universally, when talking to people trying to dial in that ultimate body, or anyone in high-stress situations for that matter, they tell me they have sleep issues. Sleep disruption is directly related to obesity and general poor health for several reasons. A couple of important reasons in the particular case we have been discussing are the changes in leptin and ghrelin kinetics. Leptin, as an appetite suppressant hormone, tends to stop working in sleep deprivation and ghrelin, the road rage hormone (give me some food or someone dies!), tends to skyrocket. As part of the whole program outlined here, keeping these hormones working properly should be a top priority.

There are many different versions of sleep disorders and disruptions with several potential causes. I have found two classic scenarios that tend to occur following (or during) a Fat to Fit lifestyle. There are, of course, many different versions of what I am about to describe, even cross-over between these two patterns, but these are the stories/scenarios that present at my office:

1. When they finally get to bed, they fall asleep before their head hits the pillow. Unfortunately, they then wake up sometime between 1:00 a.m. and 4:00 a.m. and cannot get back to sleep. It is not a groggy wake-up either. It's an "I am fully awake" wake-up (but they still feel fatigued!)

2. When this type of person crawls into bed, tired as can be, they lie there and stare at the ceiling, the walls, the underside of their pillow, the back of a face mask, etc. They cannot fall asleep, or they go in and out of N1 and N2 throughout the night (see below). This pattern continues until about 4:00 or 5:00 a.m., when they finally fall asleep, only to be disturbed shortly thereafter by their preset alarm clock.

I will refer to each of these as **Pattern 1** and **Pattern 2** later, so you know what I am talking about and how to fix it. Both patterns cause extreme duress, and fatigue all day long. Both patterns seem to have a racing mind component, or an "I cannot turn it off, doc" aspect that is very disturbing.

Both patterns also have similar physiologic and hormonal reasons behind them, and because there is a lot of alternating between the two patterns (meaning, you can fall into Pattern 1 for a while, then get into Pattern 2, or have a combination of both), the intervention is similar. I am avoiding the strict medical definitions of insomnia here, as I want to make this practical and usable. Before we get to that, let's cover some sleep facts so the "fix" makes more sense.

## Sleep Architecture

The number of hours you sleep is very important, but even more important is the quality of sleep you experience, and when you get it. It's the quality of sleep that affects your emotional, mental, cognitive, and physical well-being. If I were to pick the number of hours most people need to sleep, at the very least for *RecoverMe*, I would suggest seven hours. All age groups and walks of life have suggested hours of sleep (kids need more, etc.), but with our current crazy, busy lifestyles, if the sleep is quality—seven hours is sufficient for most people. Too much sleep is as harmful as too little sleep, so shoot for seven hours every night.

I am sure you are familiar with the old saying "An hour of sleep before midnight, is more beneficial than two hours after midnight." This is very true as when you sleep in the sun/daylight cycle is just as important.

We imagine (maybe dream is a better word here?), that sleep is when our bodies shut down. Nothing could be further from the truth. Your brain goes into full gear, your body goes into repair mode, and the amount of biologic/metabolic activity that occurs is very impressive. You just don't know it.

Your body goes through a few stages of sleep. These stages are circadian controlled, similar to and involving your hormones, and they really help dictate how you function. Each stage of sleep has very important characteristics that help you recover from overexercising and undereating and are important enough for me to mention in this context.

Quiet sleep, also known as non-REM sleep (NREM), which has three stages in it, and rapid eye movement (REM) or dreaming sleep. Quiet or deep sleep restores the body (repair and recovery) and REM sleep re-establishes the brain (emotional balance, learning, memory, etc.). Classification of the sleep stages has changed recently, so you may be familiar with Stage 1, Stage 2, and Stage 3 sleep followed by REM sleep. It is basically the same, so please do not let the small details distract you from the material.

The three stages of non-REM sleep are as follows:

- N1
    - 0 This is the initial stage of sleep, when you are slowly falling to sleep. Your muscles start to relax, your temperature drops, and your brain starts to "float." In this stage of sleep, you are easily awakened, and tend to feel drowsy and really angry if someone or something wakes you up. This usually lasts for only a few minutes before you slip into stage N2.

- N2
  - 0 N2 is the first part of "real" sleep. Everything from the neck down slows down, including your breathing, your heart rate, your temperature, etc. From the neck up, your brain starts to recollect the day, making/storing memories. You are asleep, but outside influences are realized by the brain so a noisy environment, the TV still on, your kids sneaking in after their curfew, etc. will be recognized/heard by the brain, even though you do not necessarily wake up. As you cycle through these stages (see below) you spend about half of your time sleeping in this stage.

- N3
  - o This is also called deep sleep or slow-wave sleep. Your body completely relaxes, breathing rate becomes very regular, and your pulse and blood pressure drop to roughly 30% of their waking levels. When you hit this stage, it is difficult for you to wake up, so if your kids time it correctly, they would wait until they know you are in this stage of sleep to sneak back into their rooms. Your brain then redirects blood flow to itself and gets to work. Hormones such as growth hormone (GH) get released, and your brain triggers endorphins to activate the immune system—rebuilding your army, if you will.
  - 0 If you are a younger Fat to Fit survivor, you (normally) should spend about 20% of your night in this stage of sleep. If you are older, the time spent in this stage is greatly diminished, to the point of nil if you are older than 65.

REM sleep occurs about 3 to 5 times during the night—roughly every 90 minutes. Initially, it's for a very short period, but becomes longer throughout the night. Dreaming occurs during this sleep, as your brain processes things. Your temperature comes up a little, as do your heart rate and blood pressure. Your sympathetic nervous system goes into high gear at this point, unless it has been fried by your overenthusiastic body achievement program. This sleep and activity restores and refreshes the brain—a ctrl-alt-delete if you will, as irrelevant information is cleared. Your daytime ability to think abstractly is reliant on this stage of sleep. That is why it is better to get a good night's sleep before a test, children, than to stay up all night and cram. During REM sleep your energy storage units get refilled in your body and brain, and your muscles literally go limp for the only real rest they will get.

Throughout the night, in a normal situation (not a night of anyone under a lot of stress including a Fat to Fit diet and exercise program user), you move between these stages of sleep in a very regular pattern. Deep sleep occurs in the first half of the night, and REM progressively increases until you awaken. Again—as you get older—you get less N3 sleep and more N1 sleep, with more awakenings. This is one reason why, if you are older, you get into trouble faster and with more vigor than you would have when you were in your twenties by over doing it with exercise and crazy eating.

## Sleep Pathology

Sleep disturbances, lack of sleep, poor initiation of sleep, terrible sleep maintenance, tossing-and-turning, ceiling studying, mind racing—the descriptive terms to describe sleep problems in our modern society could likely take an entire book—and many a book has been written about them! Without question, the number of people reporting to their doctor's office for some help with sleep continues to grow. As with the rest of this book, I will focus on the Fat to

Fit reasons for rotten sleep, rather than cover all the other potential reasons you sleep horribly.

Referring to what I said in the beginning of the chapter, I will classify sleep disturbance in two ways:

**Pattern 1:** When you finally get to bed, you fall asleep before your head hits the pillow and then wake up sometime between 1:00 a.m. and 4:00 a.m. and cannot get back to sleep.

**Pattern 2:** You go to bed exhausted, but cannot fall asleep until about 4:00 or 5:00 a.m., and when you finally do fall asleep, your alarm clock goes off.

**Pattern 1**

I call this pattern of sleep the *crash and roll* sleep. One tends to crash quickly, then toss, turn and roll to the point of giving up and getting up sometime between 1:00 and 4:00 a.m. This is a hormone issue. This is a jacked-up cortisol/HPA axis issue. Your killer exercise and lack of nutrients, as well as your "legal speed" to keep you going all day makes you crash really hard at night, but the hormonal disarray then wakes you in the middle of the night. Cortisol is at fault here, but also to blame is the damage done to the brain and its ability to dampen the cortisol effect at that time of night. Cortisol naturally rises at night starting around 1:00 or 2:00 a.m., but your brain is supposed to ignore it until light hits your eyes. The damage done by overexercising and undereating as professed by so many programs, not to mention just plain high stress, inhibits this.

The result is not enough sleep. This translates into poor recovery, inability to lose weight/fat, cognitive problems, emotional issues—the list goes on. What does your personal trainer, your friend at the gym, or any diet and exercise program tell you to do at this point if not losing weight or burning fat? Exercise harder, eat less and therefore sleep less—here we go again. We are not only compounding the issue at this point, but making it grow exponentially.

When you have this pattern of sleep, no matter what your age, you are sleeping like an 80-year-old going between N1 and N2 sleep, hardly any N3 sleep, and very short, sporadic REM sleep. Not good for recovery or anything else for that matter.

**Pattern 2**

Pattern 2 sleep is like a medically-diagnosable sleep disorder called delayed sleep phase disorder (DSPD). It is also called circadian rhythm sleep disorder, delayed sleep phase type. DSPD is characterized by an inability to fall asleep, even though the clock tells you it is time for bed. Studies have shown that if you could convince the rest of your life (your boss, your kids, your kids' school, store hours, etc.), to go to bed at 2:00 a.m. and wake up at 9:00 a.m. like you do—you would do great!

Since life is usually not that accommodating, Pattern 2 or DSPD is a problem. Why does this occur? If you have a teenager at home, you may be convinced they have this disease. They do, but that is because melatonin is released later in a teenager than in an old guy like me. If you recently developed this sleep pattern (but you are not a teenager), you have circadian issues brought on by your "healthy" lifestyle. All of the pathophysiology, medical studies, and specialized testing I discussed above will indirectly point you to this disorder. The exercise and diet program jacked up your hormones, and now your sleep cycle is screwed up. The fix? Take a guess!

There are several variations of these two sleep patterns and a few other actual medical diagnoses I could list here, but your doctor should be able to rule out those conditions or, at the very least, refer you to someone who can make those diagnoses if the things I suggest in this *entire book* do not work. (I emphasized "entire book" to make the point that to fix your sleep, you need to stop the Fat to Fit exercise, dieting, and supplements, eat and exercise as suggested in the book, and see your doctor for the medical portion of it).

I could go on with more than you ever need to know about sleep, but in the context of what we have covered so far, let's get to the point and get you sleeping better!

**Fixing the Sleep Issues**

The *RecoverMe* program is the solution for a good night's sleep. The combination of proper exercise, stress control via meditation and relaxation, optimization of hormones, limiting toxic exposure, controlling oxidative stress, gut health, and proper supplementation all combine to help you sleep. That's when you recover. That's when you feel better. That is when you lose weight for good, if that's your goal. Not before. Sleep has to be good for all those things to happen.

I am going to give you a list of supplements and drugs to talk to your doctor about to help you sleep. I am also going to list a few drugs you should **NEVER** use for sleep, as they just cause more issues later in life. But first—let me start with a list of things to do around sleep, like we did with eating in Chapter 10, as our goal is the big picture of overall health. This could also be called sleep hygiene, as it is behavioral and environmental training that is intended to promote better quality sleep.

**Things to do BEFORE going to bed**

**Sleep environment**

Your sleep environment must be perfect for you to sleep. You must do a few things to optimize your body's ability to sleep and here is the list with brief explanations:

1. **Make your bed every morning.** Once again, mom was right. Making your bed actually helps you sleep. For whatever reason, studies show that this simple action improves sleep.

2. **Go to bed and wake up the same time every day, even on weekends.** A tough one, but if your schedule allows for it, you will train your circadian rhythm to adjust to your schedule, not the other way around.

3. **Keep your room clean and de-cluttered.** A neat/clean sleeping environment/room is essential to your ability to fall asleep. Why this is, is also debated, but it seems to hold true.

4. **Mattress and Pillow.** Your mattress should be changed/replaced every 5–8 years, possibly more often if you are older than 40. Your favorite pillow, slobber stains and all, needs to be replaced every 2 years at max. In the interim, keep your mattress and pillows clean, using hot water for pillows and mattress covers, and then running them through the dryer on high heat to kill dust mites at least every few weeks, if not more often. For your mattress, use baking soda to suck up moisture and vacuum it off after it has sat for a day. Do this at least once a quarter.

5. **Get the correct sheets.** Do you like smooth and silky, or a little more rough and fuzzy? Silk sheets vs flannel sheets. I love silk sheets. My wife loves flannel sheets. Certainly not grounds for a divorce, as a compromise is needed and you need to find the best feeling sheets for you, for a good night's rest. A sheet is not just a sheet. That is no bull-sheet.

6. **Make your sleeping area a special place**. You may have heard the adage that the bedroom should only be used for two things: sleep and sex/procreation. Well—it is true. Get rid of computers, TVs, and other distractions. If your room is bright red or yellow, with posters of Aliens on the walls— change it. Choose calming and warm colors for your walls, blankets, etc. If you are familiar with *The Far Side* cartoon

by Gary Larsen, you may recall the cartoon where a frazzled looking bird in a cage is being covered with a blanket (over the cage) by his owner. The bird looks terrible and terrified, with most of his feathers gone, and a look of utter discontent on his face, as the blanket has all sorts of predators, such as angry-looking wolves, lions, and bears as decoration. This cartoon could not be more accurate. Make your sleeping environment a safe sanctuary.

7. **Sound proof your sleeping room.** Your brain still hears sounds when you're sleeping. Recall our smart vs. dumb teenager sneaking in after curfew. Noises, even when you do not wake up, can shift or change your sleep pattern or stage. Your sensitivity to noise and the type of noise also matter. If you drive to work in bumper-to-bumper traffic every day, a car horn may drive you batty at night and bring you right out of a deep sleep. If this is the case—sound proof your room from car noises. Think about the noises that are likely to disrupt sleep and do your best (find a way) to limit, if not completely remove them, while you are sleeping. You will still wake up if the sound is relevant to you. For example, a mother of a newborn baby can sleep through her husband's snoring, but the second that baby peeps…she is up! Getting a fan for some white noise is a great way to distract your brain from outside noises that could change your sleeping.

8. **Make a sleep diary.** One may want to consider a sleep diary to keep track of the things listed below and see if there are any obvious patterns that develop, or show up, that you could modify to improve your sleep. There are apps now that do a lot of this for you. Your sleep diary should contain statements about:

- Bedtime and time you get up
- Awakenings and why you woke up
- Time in bed vs. time sleeping
- Did you fall asleep or take a nap during the day
- Any special events that may have changed your sleep patterns
- Any exposure to drugs or medication

There are also sleep questionnaires (Epworth and Stanford Sleepiness Scale) available to help you classify your sleep if you are interested.

9. **Make your room as dark as possible and start dimming your room lights as you prepare for bed.** Light and darkness have massive control over your circadian clock. If you have an artificially well-lit room, it will be tougher to get to sleep. As the sun sets, melatonin in your brain starts to be released, telling the brain and body it is about time for bed. Bright light, especially artificial light, stops this. Make sure you have low-wattage incandescent lights in your room. If you are one who gets up at night to pee, make sure you have little night lights to prevent you from turning on a bright overhead light. Get dark shades for the windows and order them two sizes larger than you may need, so they stop light from sneaking around corners and waking you up.

    a. A common theme among couples with sleep dilemmas is, "She is a night owl, I am a morning person. We cannot coordinate our time in bed, and I know that is part of the problem." Drugs are, of course, one option (taking drugs and/or drugging the other person), as is good sleep hygiene, as discussed here. An interesting study done at the University of Colorado in Boulder showed that our propensity to be night owls or early birds can be adjusted by exposure to natural light, that is, sunlight. We all have a natural circadian rhythm that balances directly in relation to sunlight. The study demonstrated that if one is exposed to sunrise/sunset light as it occurs via nature, and not exposed to modern conveniences and lights, early birds and night owls sync their sleep patterns to this everyday occurrence. What this means to you night owls who have a heck of a time waking up in the morning is that it would do you wonders to get up and expose yourself to as much sunlight as possible. Then, in the evening, limit electric lights, screen time, and even personal electronic devices that blare with the intensity of the sun. This will start to override your propensity to stay up late, as the hormones responsible for your circadian rhythm adjust. It will also allow for a better night's rest and correspond to a more wakeful and alert day. Once again, the power of all-natural living, limiting screen time, and simplicity override modern answers and temporary solutions.

10. **Keep your room cool at night.** Expert opinion seems to be that the ideal room temperature for sleep is 65 degrees. A room that is too hot disrupts your natural cooling mechanism that helps prepare you for sleep. Some studies suggest that certain forms of insomnia are dysregulation of body temperature—one does not cool down as one should at night and it keeps you awake. A small study at the National Institutes of Health has shown that turning down the thermostat a few notches at night may expand brown fat tissue mass and activity and, thereby, create a fat burning environment while sleeping. Brown fat tissue also improves insulin

sensitivity and glucose metabolism, so this may be of some benefit to people with insulin resistance and diabetes, as well. Sleeping in an environment that is too warm (e.g., the thermostat in the 70s or higher, multiple blankets on the bed, and/or an electric or heating blanket or device) did not produce this added fat burning and metabolic effect.

11. **Make your sleeping area smell good.** Smells, good and bad, can affect or influence your dreams and help you doze off every night. For example, lavender has been shown to lower blood pressure and heart rate and get you into a relaxed state for sleep. If your husband ate Taco Bell before bed, his smell alone may change your ability to sleep and, at the very least, give you nightmares. Make sure your sleeping area smells good.

12. **Do not eat or drink before bed. If you do, make it the correct food.** Ideally, one never eats a few hours before bed. This is more difficult if you are following Track 2 in the 5:2 MDC for the *RecoverMe* eating plan, so it will take some experimenting. Never drink alcohol before bed. You may think you sleep better, but with alcohol in your system, you never get into the important deep stages of sleep. If you do eat before bed, make it a light meal with good protein and clean carbs. The amino acid tryptophan, found in most protein sources, can help with sleep if the amounts are small. Carbohydrates increase insulin, which increases serotonin in the brain and may help you sleep better. Believe it or not, but a potato works well for sleep. You must decide however, what is more beneficial for your goals and *RecoverMe*? Eating before bed to get better sleep, or not eating before bed to optimize anabolic and fat burning hormones?

13. **Do not exercise before bed.** If your schedule allows it, get a few hours of rest before going to bed. Exercise gets all the stimulant hormones running and, in some people, they are slow to slow down.

14. **Nap on a regular basis.** A 20-minute nap will increase alertness and concentration, and even improve your mood. A longer nap, though, and you may very well wake up during the wrong phase of your sleep cycle and feel groggy and tired.

15. **Avoid tobacco, alcohol, MSG, artificial sweeteners, and exercise at least a few hours before it's your fall asleep time.** These things are activating, and may greatly influence your ability to fall asleep. If your only time to exercise is after work before bed, utilize Holy Basil following exercise will help lower cortisol and allow for better sleep. (Reviewed in Chapter 9)

16. **Stop all handheld electronics when the sun goes down.** I saved this for last, as it is the one you are least likely to listen to or do. Before I tell you why, let me tell you about a few patients of mine with refractory insomnia. After every drug was tried, sleep studies galore, and even some experimental drugs attempted, the thing that helped my patients in this situation sleep better was getting rid of their cell phones at night. It's true. Handheld electronics emit a blue light in the 460-nanometer range of the electromagnetic spectrum. This blue light stops melatonin, the sleep hormone, from being released. Your brain thinks it's high noon. Handheld electronics are right near your face. Not good for those of you needing a good night's rest. Ideally, when the sun goes down, you tell all of your friends and family to use the old-fashioned land line to call you. That is

hard if you live where I do. In January the sun goes down at 4:30 p.m.! So ideally, put your handheld electronics away a few hours before bed, and never read from one in bed (Kindle causes insomnia!).

Now that you have the proper set up for a good night's *RecoverMe* sleep, let me review the basic hormonal/physiological needs to obtain a good night's rest and then provide you with some solutions. As there are some drugs your doctor may suggest/prescribe that should NEVER be used for sleep or any *RecoverMe* program, I will mention those first, then follow it with some supplements and drugs that may have a role in helping you sleep and recover from your Fat to Fit to Fat program.

## Basic Sleep Chemistry

To fall asleep, you must have melatonin and GABA present and elevated while there is a concurrent drop in cortisol and glutamate. Melatonin is produced by a gland in the back of the brain called the Pineal gland (the gland gets its name because it is shaped like a pinecone). The pineal gland is turned on by darkness and turned off by light—it follows the sun. Melatonin helps determine your circadian rhythm by inducing sleep-wake cycles and controlling blood pressure, and it is a strong antioxidant. GABA or gamma-aminobutyric acid is the primary inhibitory hormone of the brain. You must have GABA present for non-REM sleep. GABA also inhibits the release of cortisol by stopping cortisol-releasing hormone (CRH) from the hypothalamus. Something we briefly touch on a few chapters ago. Glutamate is the primary excitatory neurotransmitter in the brain. I will mention B vitamins in the suggested supplement section, and one of the primary reasons is vitamin B6 is required to convert glutamate to GABA (excitatory to inhibitory). As with all hormonal interplays, you can see a fine balance that must be obtained to get proper and good sleep.

Many of the supplements I am about to mention and the prescription drugs that may play a short-term role in helping you get a better night rest all work on three primary sleep related hormones: Cortisol, Melatonin, and GABA. Here is a simple chart to help you see what the hormones should ideally be doing for you to get a good night sleep:

| Hormone | Sleep Induction | Sleep Maintenance |
|---|---|---|
| Cortisol | ⬇ | ⬆ The excitatory effect on the brain should normally be blocked or dampened. When this fails, Pattern 1 sleep disturbance occurs. |
| GABA | ⬆ | ⬆⬇ |
| Melatonin | ⬆⬇ | ⬆ |

## Prescription and Over-the-Counter Drugs You Should Avoid like the Plague!

There is a very common drug class prescribed by medical providers for poor sleep and the anxiety that comes from any high-stress situation. These drugs are benzodiazepines, such as Valium (Zentran), Lorazepam (Ativan), Alprazolam (Xanax), Clonazepam (Klonopin), Temazopam (Restoril), etc.

Benzodiazepines (benzos) are a class of drugs that work on the brain, acting selectively on gamma-aminobutyric acid-A (GABA-A receptors in the brain. GABA is a neurotransmitter that inhibits or reduces the activity of nerve cells. It is your primary inhibitory or relaxing brain hormone. All benzodiazepines work in a similar way, but there are differences in how long they affect you. Valium, for example, has a half-life of 72 hours, and shorter acting ones, such as Ativan, have a half-life one-third of that. The problem is that these are VERY addictive. After a few doses, you can't fall asleep without them. They decrease slow wave sleep and REM sleep. They have been linked to increased falls and injury in the elderly, memory problems, and even dementia, if you use them long enough. As we are trying to fix things here, these drugs are the last things you want to use, as your problems will just get worse!

Another set of drugs you should avoid include over-the-counter antihistamines such as diphenhydramine (Benadryl) products. Antihistamines decrease sleep latency. Tylenol PM and knock-offs of this drug fit this category. Similar drugs in this class you should avoid include doxylamine and hydroxyzine. These are all also used to treat allergies as well.

Antihistamines such as diphenhydramine (Benadryl), hydroxyzine, and doxylamine inhibit a primary brain activating hormone, histamine. Kicking histamine out of play causes day-time fatigue and severe hangovers that may last for days. It compounds over time. If you're reading this, you are already likely fatigued and begging for energy—why would you make it worse in the attempt to get better?

Old antidepressants called tricyclic antidepressants such as amitriptyline (Elavil), imipramine (Tofranil), and doxepin (Sinequan) (there are many others), should also be avoided. They suppress REM sleep. They work on several of your brains neurotransmitters and all of them are associated with weight gain over time (why did you start that intense diet and exercise program in the first place?) Trazadone, one I will discuss in a few paragraphs, falls into this category, but tends to not cause the weight gain or suppress REM sleep as the others do.

Many antipsychotics (Zyprexa, Seroquel, and others) and antiepileptic (Neurontin and Lyrica) drugs are also used for sleep. Avoid these as well. They have a side effect profile longer than your leg, including weight gain.

Avoid these drugs at all cost. They just compound your problem.

# Drugs and Supplements for Pattern 1

As a review, Pattern 1 is the person who falls right to sleep, but then wakes up in the middle of the night.

This is a true hormone problem. High-stress situations such as overexercising and undereating with continuously elevated sympathetic tone and high cortisol are the issues at hand here. As I mentioned in my description of REM sleep, the sympathetic (fight or flight) system is very active in this stage of sleep. If you are constantly in a high state, due to your chosen activities or other stressors in life, including ones beyond your control, REM sleep does not have a rise in sympathetic expression for a couple of reasons:

1. You are already there. How can you elevate that tone if you are already there? This means a basic failure of one of the primary aspects of this stage of sleep, meaning—you don't get into this stage of sleep!

2. The nutrients needed to make the hormones responsible for sympathetic tone (amino acids such as Tyrosine), have been used up. You cannot build a house when no wood/supplies are available!

3. Your brain has lost the ability to dampen the naturally occurring rise in cortisol in the middle of the night, and you wake up.

Aspects of treatment include lowering sympathetic tone throughout the day. That means the following:

1. QUIT the yo-yo dieting and out-of-control exercise the current program you are doing has suggested you do.

2. Replace the amino acid precursors of the needed neurotransmitters with regular supplementation.

It is also essential that you fix the HPA axis and lower cortisol. This is done by:

1. QUITTING the Fat to Fit program
2. Using the supplements mentioned in Chapter 8 and Chapter 11 to help balance cortisol and DHEA
3. RELAXING as often as possible. Take a yoga or stretching class. Meditate and pray whenever you can. Spend time outdoors in the sun and absorb the sounds of nature. If you're in a bad relationship—get out or get help!

As far as prescription drugs that may be of benefit if you are a Pattern 1 person, you need something to help you maintain sleep. Drugs like Ambien and Lunesta help initiate sleep, but with this pattern, you will wake up at your usual early 1:00 to 4:00 a.m. waking time. You need something like Trazadone, an old antidepressant that works on multiple brain hormones, to help you maintain your sleep. Trazadone is a powerful drug and you need to discuss its use in great detail with your doctor, so you understand side effects, interactions, reactions, etc. A low dose is all that is needed. Like most drugs, side effects are dose-dependent. If you are on the supplements I am suggesting, have quit the stupidity of the Fat to Fit program, are following the eating plan and lighter exercise schedule, the addition of this drug can be of great use—in the short term. Fix the problem and get off the drug.

**Here is a chart of supplements and drugs for a Pattern 1 insomniac:**

| Supplement/Drug | Dose | Time of day to take it | How long to take it | What it does |
|---|---|---|---|---|
| Zinc/Magnesium/B6 combo products | 30/450/10 mg for men 20/300/6 mg for women | Before bed | As needed | Provides essential sleep nutrients |
| Vitamin C | 2000–3000 mg | Once a day | Lifetime | Helps fix the HPA axis |
| B-complex | 1 dose | Twice a day | Lifetime | Helps fix the HPA axis. Converts Glutamate to GABA |
| 5-HTP (slow release) | 50–100 mg | Before bed | Three to six months | Precursor to serotonin |
| L-Theanine | 200–400 mg | Up to four times a day | As needed | Calming agent. Increases GABA |
| Relora | 250 mg | Three times a day | Three to six months | Lowers cortisol |
| Phosphorylated Serine (Seriphos®) | 1–2 tablets | Before bed | Three to six months | Lowers cortisol levels in the brain |
| Rhodiola | 100–200 mg | Twice a day—breakfast and lunch, and if needed, before bed | Three to six months | Adaptogenic compound |
| Melatonin | 3–6 mg | 1–2 hours before bed | Three to six months | Strong antioxidant and sleep aid |
| DRUG: Trazadone | 25–50 mg | Before bed | Three to six months | Medication that helps you maintain sleep |
| DRUG: Micronized Progesterone | 25–100 mg for a woman and 5–20 mg for a man (oral is best) | Before bed | Three to six months | Increases GABA |

I have covered most of these supplements/drugs already, so in this section of the book, I will just review the drugs I have not discussed yet.

## Progesterone

Progesterone is the hormone of pregnancy: pro-gestation = progesterone. Western medicine considers it just that, with the additional action of causing the endometrium (uterine lining) to sluff off once a month, e.g., menstruation. As a quick review: in the first portion of the menstrual cycle (follicular phase), the uterine lining builds up waiting for a fertilized egg to implant. If a fertilized egg does not implant, in the second phase of the menstrual cycle (luteal phase), estrogen decreases and progesterone causes the lining to fall off. This causes menstrual bleeding.

When considering progesterone for sleep and as an antianxiety drug you need to make sure it is God-made progesterone, **NOT** progestin, the artificial progesterone. Unfortunately, most medical providers do not know the difference between progesterone and progestin. Artificial progestin, such as medroxyprogesterone acetate (Provera), is a horrible drug responsible for everything from hormonal disruption, increased cancer risk, insulin resistance, and many other issues that should concern you if you are taking it! This is NOT the progesterone I am talking about. I am talking about the bio-identical hormone made by big pharm called micronized progesterone (Prometrium), or compounded by a bio-identical hormone pharmacy.

Progesterone does so much more than just being involved in pregnancy or menstruation! It is a neuro-steroid that is converted to Allopregnanolone in the brain, which then stimulates GABA, the inhibitory neurotransmitter I already discussed. Just like the addictive and bad-for-you benzodiazepines, progesterone works on the same chemical needed for relaxation/sleep in the brain, without the bad side-effects! In my experience, it is the best sleep aid and antianxiety drug out there for women!

Men, too, can benefit from progesterone usage. Why would a man need/use a hormone of pregnancy? Don't worry—he won't get pregnant! In men with refractory or hard to treat insomnia, progesterone does wonders. It is a great go-to when all else has failed and when I am worried about a man's long-term health and the consequences of my prescription writing. On a side note, several AAS are progesterone-based (I am certainly not promoting the use of AAS), so it has been tested for you by others. Men have been using those for years, and although these have many side effects beyond the scope of this book (sperm production, etc.), it goes to show that they can be used in men without problems related to the progesterone nature of the drug.

## Melatonin

Melatonin is produced by a gland in the back of the brain called the pineal gland (the gland gets its name because it is shaped like a pinecone). The pineal gland is turned on by darkness, and turned off by light—it follows the sun. This is why using handheld electronic devices before bed is not a good idea. The pineal gland thinks it's high noon when you are staring at those contraptions and does not release melatonin. Melatonin helps determine your circadian rhythm by inducing sleep-wake cycles and controlling blood pressure, and it is a strong antioxidant. Using melatonin, with all the other suggested interventions, can be a great adjunct to your sleep. There are some drug/melatonin interactions so talk to your doctor before using it. Dosage ranges from 1 to 20 mg and it should be taken at least an hour (in some cases more) before lying down to sleep. I suggest the lower ranges of dosing as higher (greater than 10 mg) is likely to cause a hangover the next day.

There are a couple of prescription melatonin agonists available including a controlled release version and one called Ramelteon (Rozerem). You could also talk to your doctor about having it compounded—for example a mix of immediate and controlled release melatonin.

## L-Theanine

L-Theanine is the ingredient in green tea that makes you appreciate green tea. It is very calming, as it directly stimulates the production of alpha brain waves, causing deep relaxation. It also increases brain derived neurotropic factor or BDNF. BDNF enhances neurotransmitter function and enhances neurogenesis and plasticity. It also works in the formation of GABA, the primary inhibitory neurotransmitter. Doses are 100–400 mg up to three times a day for anxiety and wrecked nerves, and 40 min before sleep.

## Rhodiola

Rhodiola is an adaptogenic compound that helps to decrease the brain's response to cortisol in the middle of the night. I prefer to use this one in the day time—breakfast and lunch, but for those with really bad Pattern 1 sleep issues, I would give it a try at night. There are several studies on this one in athletes and recovery, especially after vigorous exercise.

## 5-HTP

5-Hydroxytryptophan (5-HTP), not to be confused with 5-hydroxytryptamine or serotonin (5-HT), is a precursor, as well as a metabolic intermediate, in the creation of the neurotransmitter serotonin. It has several uses in alternative medicine including being used as an appetite suppressant, antidepressant, and (why it's mentioned here) a sleep aid as serotonin is the precursor for melatonin. Serotonin is essential for good sleep. Let me give you an example that I would bet 10:1 you already knew. Do you sleep better when you have milk and cookies or a bowl of cereal before bed? You do. The reason is because carbs raise serotonin. Serotonin also crashes, which is why you go back and have more cookies or ice cream, or whatever your sweetie is, as your brain is begging for more serotonin!

Taking the precursor for serotonin gives the brain the ability to make more and do all the things listed above, including a good night's rest. These is slow-acting and quick-acting. If you are a

Pattern 1 sleeper, you want the long or slow-acting version—50 to 100 mg before your bedtime. If you are a Pattern 2 sleeper, a short or quick-acting version would be best. Dose is 100–150 mg before your bedtime.

5-HTP has a number of drug interactions, so be sure to talk to your doctor before this one is used!

## Phosphorylated Serine (Seriphos®)

This brand name supplement decreases cortisol at bed time to help decrease awakening throughout the night. This supplement can make some people feel bad if their cortisol is already too low from chronic stress. It is a good idea to do a diurnal salivary cortisol test with your doctor before trying this one.

## Zinc/Magnesium/B6 combo products

This combo of supplements has been used in the physique world for years. Each of these minerals and vitamins has unique properties that may help users get into deeper sleep. How this is effective is only speculation, but my guess would be, especially due to the crowd that promotes it, that poor sleep quality can be partly to blame for nutrient/mineral deficiencies. Replace them, and you sleep better. That is why this is a great supplement for sleep for the Fat to Fit to Fat crowd—you're deficient in these, as we have already discussed! Doses vary, but it appears the best dose for men is 30 mg of zinc, 450 mg of magnesium, and 10 mg of B6. Women should take a 20-mg dose of zinc, 300 mg of magnesium, and 6 mg of B6.

There is a whole list of other sleep aids you could consider trying. I did not include them here, as I do not use them as often as I do the ones mentioned above. These would include things such as Valerian, Passionflower, Lemon Balm, and Lavender. Talk to your doctor or natural practitioner as to which one of those may be best for you.

**Drugs and Supplements for Pattern 2**

As a review, Pattern 2 is the person who cannot fall asleep, no matter what they do, until it's close to time to get up!

Pattern 2 people need to initiate sleep so this is what needs to be done:

1. Do the right things during the day, including everything mentioned so far in this book.

    a. Everything a Pattern 1 person needs to do

2. Become calm BEFORE going to bed, with all the suggestions on sleep hygiene above. It also is of great benefit for Pattern 2 sleepers to meditate before crawling into bed.

3. Make the right environment (light, sound, smells, sheets, etc.) for sleep, as mentioned above

4. Utilize some supplements and drugs during the day and, if needed, before bed

## Here is a chart of supplements and drugs for a Pattern 2 insomniac:

| Supplement/Drug | Dose | Time of day to take it | How long to take it | What it does |
|---|---|---|---|---|
| L-Tyrosine | 1000 mg | Twice a day | Three to six months | Provides the precursor amino acid for production of neurotransmitters |
| Vitamin C | 2000–3000 mg | Once a day | Three to six months | Helps fix the HPA axis |
| B-complex | 1 dose | Twice a day | Three to six months | Helps fix the HPA axis. Converts Glutamate to GABA |
| L-Theanine | 200–400 mg | Up to four times a day | As needed | Calming agent Increases GABA |
| Relora | 250 mg | Three times a day | Three to six months | Lowers cortisol |
| Melatonin | 3–6 mg | 1–2 hours before bed | Three to six months | Strong antioxidant and sleep aid |
| 5-HTP (fast release) | 100–150 mg | Before bed | Three to six months | Precursor to serotonin |
| Zinc/Magnesium/B6 combo products | 30/450/10 for men 20/300/6 for women | Before bed | As needed | Provides essential sleep nutrients |
| DRUG: Ambien | 5–10 mg | Before bed | One to two months | Medication that helps you initiate sleep |
| DRUG: Lunesta | 2–3 mg | Before bed | One to two months | Medication that helps you initiate sleep |
| DRUG: Xyrem | 4.5 grams | Before bed | One to two months | Medication that helps you initiate sleep |
| DRUG: Micronized Progesterone | 25–100 mg for a woman and 5–20 mg for a man (oral is best) | Before bed | Three to six months | Increases GABA |

I have covered most of these supplements/drugs already, so in this section of the book, I will just review the drugs I have not discussed yet. Of note, these drugs should not be used together. I am listing them here so you are aware of them for a good discussion with your doctor. **NEVER** use these ***drugs together***. These drugs all have serious side effects, so **DO NOT** take them without first having a good discussion with your doctor. Ideally, you avoid these drugs as they all have some potential concerns. I am adding them here, as the goal of this book is to arm you with the information to get better following your wild attempts to get a better body. If you do utilize them, never use them for more than one month at a time. Hopefully, with the information found in this book, you fix yourself and no longer need these chemicals.

## The Z-Drugs (Nonbenzodiazepine Hypnotics)

### Ambien (Zolpidem)

Ambien (Zolpidem) is a sedative/hypnotic that is a short-acting nonbenzodiazepine that increases the activity of GABA. This means it acts like a benzo, but may not (and I emphasize **MAY** not) have the same long-term side effects as a benzodiazepine. It acts within 15 minutes of taking it and will help initiate sleep. Important warning: if you do not do everything I have talked about in this chapter and you take this drug, you will wake up four hours after taking it, and your problems will not only be unsolved, they will worsen! It is good for short-term use, to help you recover from a Pattern 2 sleep disorder involving a Fat to Fit program.

### Lunesta (Eszopiclone)

Lunesta is also a sedative/hypnotic that is a short-acting non-benzodiazepine that modifies the activity of GABA. Just like Ambien, it **MAY** not have the same long-term side effects of a benzodiazepine. It acts within minutes of taking it and will help initiate sleep. Important warning: if you do not do everything I have talked about in this chapter and you take this drug, you will wake up four hours after taking it, and your problems will not only not be solved, the will worsen! It is good for short-term use, to help you recover from a Pattern 2 sleep disorder.

## Central Nervous System Depressant

### Xyrem (Sodium Oxybate)

Xyrem is a gamma hydroxybutyrate (GHB) drug that is a powerful central nervous system depressant. You may recognize the name GHB from media reports, as it has been used as a date-rape drug by less than decent people. It knocks you out really quickly, and may be a useful adjunct for severe Pattern 2 people. It has a ton of potential side effects and writing a prescription for this drug requires a ton of paperwork and effort by your doctor. You should consult a sleep specialist for this one, as most primary care doctors would not touch it with a ten-foot pole! In the short term, with all the interventions mentioned so far, it can get your sleep back on track, but you only should take it for a limited/short time.

### Other Potential Interventions

Cognitive behavior therapy is also another potential intervention with some good data behind it. I have been really impressed with this technique for improving both Patterns 1 and 2 following a Fat to Fit program. Talk to your doctor if that sounds interesting to you.

# RECOVERME SLEEP SUMMARY

Everything I have discussed here really works. Not sleeping is becoming one of the main reasons primary care doctors are consulted on a regular basis. Sleep problems are becoming more problematic than the common cold or back pain. If you apply **EVERYTHING** I have discussed so far in this book, you have a chance to get better sleep and *RecoverMe* from your Fat to Fit program. If you have questions or variations from Patterns 1 or 2 I discussed above, talk to your doctor or email me and my team, so we can try to get a little deeper into potential problems to find your personal solution!

# CHAPTER 13
## Conclusions and FAQs

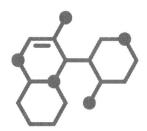

Hopefully reading or listening to this book was a little less painful than doing, completing, or suffering the after effects of a modern diet and exercise program. My goal was to give people a real answer and solution to a problem that is going viral. The pressure on every age group, in every setting and situation, to look like a super hero is hard for me to wrap my brain around. These Fat to Fit programs sneak in everywhere you turn promising you a new body and a new life **IF** you get that body (which only **THAT** particular program can provide, by-the-way). They come in every guise imaginable, but hopefully, after reading this book, you will start to recognize them all as the same product. Just sold with a slightly different twist on or approach to it, or gimmick, or device, or spokesperson, or model, or reality TV show, etc.

My expectation is that you also have the information needed to formulate your own plan in recovery. Use the information here to get better, stay better, and stay away from future Fat to Fit programs disguised as healthy or **THE** answer to your health and body goals.

I can summarize everything I hoped to accomplish with this book in a few simple statements:

- I want you to understand the pathophysiology of almost all of the diet and exercise programs out there and why you feel the way you do, and why you should forever on avoid them.

  0 Low calories and excessive exercise are the problem, not the solution to the body you want and the health you need.

- Once this was accomplished I wanted you to understand how to work with a doctor to work up the metabolic, oxidative, gut, and hormonal issues that occur following a high-stress situation and start to get them fixed.

- I want you to understand how to prepare and then recover properly for and from exercise. Then use the proper "smart" exercise for the *RecoverMe* process, so you can eventually go back to the exercise of your choosing.

- The foundation of this *RecoverMe* outline after a Fat to Fit program is the eating plan. Food is medicine, and should be used as such to help optimize your health and balance your hormones (especially the lifestyle ones), and I hope you grasped that in the *RecoverMe* process, **HOW** to eat is just as important as **WHAT** to eat.

- You need to learn how to sleep. The high stress in combination with an up-to-the-minute diet and exercise program wrecks people's sleep patterns. Sleep is essential for **RecoverMe**.

- Finally—I gave you a list of some wonderful medicinal supplements and nutraceuticals that can help you on your path to wellness and feeling good. Use these wisely and be sure to check with your doctor before taking any of them.

Do not forget, 99% of the diet and exercise, weight loss, even health programs out there fall under the Fat to Fit philosophy. It's self-perpetuating and self-serving. You cannot tell me that the smart people at some of these big national programs, including the DVD sets sold on TV and the medically-based programs, are not fully aware you will eventually fail with their system and come back for more (or the latest greatest version). Of course they know this fact. That's how they make their yacht payments. You need to break out of the vicious, yet very popular, cycle you are in and get better for life. (PS: Your "body for life" is not a 12-week program. I, for one, hope to live longer than 12 weeks.)

This program I have outlined provides two primary things: 1. Help for you to heal from your efforts to get that perfect body. 2. Give you a plan for life after you get better and recover. I think it is just as important, in a true therapeutic/curative program, to maintain that "fix" once you are better. For example, although appealing in the short term, what good is it in the big picture to cure someone's cancer for one year knowing it will come back in 13 months? Are we happy with those 12 months? Of course! But would it not be better to cure it for life? That is the goal of this book. To help you gain the perspective and knowledge to maintain the look and feel and health you want until the good Lord himself tells you to leave this earth.

As it is apparent I like charts, I have included one final chart in the book, a summary chart. The summary chart puts into perspective how to proceed with healing from the common and popular diet and exercise programs, using a make-believe time schedule (in other words, you make your own schedule based on the time frame that suits you best). This chart includes the first six months. As you read in the case studies, it takes some people much longer, so extend your intervention as long as you need to, and use lab work to document objective changes as you are moving forward. I would highly encourage you to do the program in this fashion for at least six months. Nothing shorter. After six months, if you are back to your old self again, my advice is never to get involved with a Fat to Fit program again! Just live the good life. Consider possibly having a few labs checked on a yearly basis or as frequently as your primary care doctor suggests.

Of course, if you get stuck and think that I, or someone from my team, could be of assistance, contact us via the contact information at the end of the book, and we will do our best to help you figure it out!

| | Month 1 | Month 2 | Month 3 | Month 4 | Month 5 | Month 6 |
|---|---|---|---|---|---|---|
| **Medical work up/ recheck including labs, etc.** | Initial Work up – doctors visit and labs | Labs if indicated | Recheck or follow up labs for comparison to initial labs | Labs if indicated | Labs if Indicated | Recheck or follow up labs for comparison to 3-month labs |
| **Eating Plan** | MCD 5:2 | MCD 5:2 | MCD 5:2 | MCD 3:1 | MCD 3:1 | MCD 2:1 |
| **Exercise schedule** | RecoverMe Plan | RecoverMe Plan | RecoverMe Plan | Incorporate your favorite program back in slowly | Increase your favorite program | Return to regular exercise, but continue to recover properly using the information in this book! |
| **Supplements** | As suggested | As Suggested | As suggested | Start to wean off those specific to your age/sex | Stop those specific to age and sex, unless medically indicated to continue | Continue the supplements you feel are most appropriate for your situation |

I will now conclude the book with a few frequently asked ques-tions in anticipation of those that may come up while reading/listen-ing to the book. The majority of these came directly from patients after we initiated the **RecoverMe** program following a Fat to Fit plan.

This is followed by some contact information if you are interested in getting in touch with me directly for questions, a visit, a medical consult, a physique show consult, or if you would like me to present at an event you are hosting or organizing.

## FAQs

### How does alcohol fit into the recovery program?

Very common question. My suggestion is you avoid alcohol while recovering from any stressful situation, including rigorous diet and exercise for at least the first three months. As it is nothing but a toxin, and you need to clear yourself of all toxins, I would avoid it. Sugary alcohols like beer and mixed drinks, I would avoid like the plague. Have you ever met someone who brags on the fact they don't like sugar? Ask them how much beer they drink, that is, their sugar source. These beverages cause a hormonal response that is exactly the opposite of what we want while recovering. One could argue that certain alcohols, such as whiskey or vodka, may be okay, but I refer to my toxin statement above.

### You suggest exercising in the morning after getting up. I cannot exercise until evening, due to my work and family schedule. Please advise?

I get this question all the time from **Better Than Steroids** readers, too. There is plenty of evidence that exercising first thing in the morning is of great benefit. But there is more evidence that exercising when you can (or when your schedule allows) is what is most important! In other words, do it in the morning if you can. If you cannot, don't worry about it and do it when you can!

**I cannot afford all the testing you suggested. What should I do?**

I provided information on thousands of dollars' worth of testing for a couple of reasons: 1. So you would know it was available, as it is off the radar of most doctors out there. 2. To help you understand the pathophysiology that occurs in your body while doing or finishing a modern diet and exercise program. You don't need the testing to get better and fix yourself. Might you get there quicker if you had the testing? Most certainly. Can you get better without the testing, just by understanding the problem and applying the *RecoverMe* exercise, eating, and supplement plan? Again, most certainly!

**I cannot afford taking all those supplements for even a few months—suggestions?**

I refer to the above question. Yes, taking the suggested supplements helps, but the cure is in quitting and then never doing a crazy diet and/or exercise program again, lowering your cortisol, letting the lifestyle hormones balance so the other hormones can balance by following the *RecoverMe* exercise and eating plans, and once again, never doing a Fat to Fit program again!

**Dr. Willey, if you had to pick only ONE supplement to take for helping to recover from a Fat to Fit program, what would it be?**

I would, without hesitation, say magnesium. This mineral is involved with over 300 different processes in your body, including balancing pH, optimizing hormones, used in electron transport through cell membranes, co-factor for enzymes, etc. Insurance companies would be very wise if they allowed/requested everyone get an RBC Mg+ level and get everyone to a proper amount in the body.

**I cannot find a doctor who has any idea what you are talking about here. Where can I find a doctor who not only orders these tests, but understands how to interpret them?**

These tests are familiar to functional medicine doctors and antiaging doctors. How they interpret them may be different unless they really understand what excessive exercise and low calorie eating and what it does to the body. I am happy to try to help you find someone in your area who may be of assistance. Shoot me an email (see contact info).

**(Similar question to the one above) My doctor says you are a quack, and he thinks working this problem up is pointless. Any advice?**

Ha ha ha! I love that one! Without being rude right back, I would suggest they look a little further into the reason they became doctors. Most of us had the goal of helping people. That is still my goal, and this work up I suggested, the eating plan, the exercise program, and the suggested supplements do just that. It helps people. Do we have tons of medical literature and backing on all the tests? No. Does working this up and treating it fall under the auspices of evidence-based medicine or best medical practices? No. Does it work? Yes. Would this argument I just proposed stand muster in a high-school debate contest? Probably not.

Think about this: over 65% (higher by some reports) of the medicine we doctors are prescribing each day, we are using off-label. That means the FDA has **NOT** approved the medication for use in the area it is being used for. That also means no blinded-controlled trials or evidence-based medical practices behind it. How many doctors write prescriptions for dangerous antibiotics for viral infections? How often does western medicine do serious harm, over time, by keeping people on their reflux medication/acid suppressors (PPIs in particular) for more than a few days? Or for any other drug for that matter? How many in medicine know the Number Needed to Treat

(NNT)* of all the drugs they prescribe? If they did know that number, they likely would throw away their prescription pads.

I have a duck at home. Her name is Jumbo. She is hilarious. She thinks she is a chicken, as that's who she hangs out with. Your doctor can call me a quack. I am fine with it as, in my mind, he is just comparing me to Jumbo. The difference is I know I am not a chicken, even though I may be surrounded by them. After your doctor is done bashing, and you still feel horrible, call me.

***NNT or Numbers Needed to Treat** is a very important, but little-known statistic (even by doctors), that allows you to see how effective a drug is. It is the number of patients who must be treated to prevent one adverse outcome **OR** the number of patients who must be treated for one patient to benefit from the drug treatment. Needless to say, the NNT of most drugs is very high. In other words, for every person treated with drug therapy, playing Vegas odds, I would say the drug is not working. Let me give you some examples:

> Statin drugs for lowering cholesterol for primary prevention of cardiovascular disease, the NNT is greater than 100. That means you must treat over 100 people for the drug to benefit one of them.

> Nexium, the Proton Pump Inhibitor or PPI for acid reflux, 25 people must take it to get benefit for one person.

> Finasteride, a prostate drug used to help men urinate better and avoid having a surgical procedure (to urinate better), requires 39 men to use it so one of them does not wind up under the urologist's knife.

> There is one more very important fact with NNT: the people **NOT** benefited by the drug still suffer the risks and side effects of the drugs and costs of the treatment.

Guess what has an **NNT of 1**? In other words, what intervention helps **everyone** who does it? Diet, exercise, and a few of the hormones. Sounds like this *RecoverMe* program aye?

**You really push exercising in the sun. Should I worry about skin cancer?**

Another great question. Let us review some facts on skin cancer. Does the majority of skin cancer kill people (basal cell and squamous cell carcinoma)? No. Do dermatologists make a lot of money treating these cancers? Yes. Each year over 5.4 million cases of non-melanoma skin cancer are treated in more than 3.3 million people. Is there a lot of skin cancer out there? Yes, but it cannot be completely blamed on the sun. We are an aging population and our overall health is atrocious—high stress, high toxin exposure, high oxidative stress, etc. This is what causes cancer, not the sun. If your health is good, the sun is good. If your overall health is poor and mechanism of repair does not work well, the sun can be an issue. Get the big picture? Get and stay healthy and play outside as often as possible.

That being said, let's talk really quickly about sunscreens. The Environmental Working Group (www.ewg.org) (great site by-the-way to learn how your make up might be making you sick, among other things) states that 75% of sunscreens don't work. Most of them contain chemicals that are toxic to your body. That's great—something that's supposed to prevent cancer, gives me cancer via a different mechanism. If you are at risk for sun damage, go to the above-mentioned web site and find a good, non-toxic sunscreen!

**You say calories really don't matter. Why does everyone disagree with that and do nothing but push "calories-in-to-calories-out"?**

Politics. I won't spend the time or effort here to describe the things that happened in Washington post World War II, as I spent my time describing facts you have witnessed to be true and likely experienced yourself. Look it up if you're interested. The turkeys (a.k.a. lobbyists) are to blame, and money is the reason for everything that happens in Washington.

**I did a physique show, then gained a ton of weight after it. Can I use this program to get better and do another show in the future?**

Absolutely! As I see so many physique competitors and people in the gym nice and lean one week then puffy and soft a few weeks later, it actually gave me the original idea to write this book! This very program is how I have helped many, many people get back on stage—but in full health and the ability to maintain it for life. Other than the 5-10 pounds water shifts right before stage time, one can maintain a degree of leanness, and feel good year-round, once you understand the process of the Fat to Fit lie, and never fall for it again. It is about **RecoverMe**!

**I got really nauseated after taking the handful of supplements you suggested. What should I do?**

That is not uncommon. I have been cussed out a few times for it. If that occurs, I would suggest a couple of things: 1. Spread the supplements out so you are not taking too many at a time. 2. If you feel it may be one or two causing an issue, stop everything for a week, and slowly add each one back, a week at a time, to find the culprit. 3. Use online resources to compound all your supplements into powder or other delivery systems. 4. Purchase capsules of all the supplements and make your own powder drink by breaking them apart over a glass of water.

**I just like cardio. Do I have to lift weights?**

Do you have to breathe? Do you have to go to the bathroom occasionally? Yes—you **MUST** incorporate resistance training to obtain and maintain **ALL** aspects of health.

**Genetically, I am doomed to be fat and feel crappy. My mother is fat and feels crappy. My father and his brothers are fat and feel crappy. My sister just feels crappy. Do I have a chance not to be fat and to feel good?**

Unequivocally. Will you look like one of the motivational Pinterest pictures that love to call you fat, ugly, and weak? Not likely, but you never know. Genetics play a role in your health, but your lifestyle and environment play a very powerful part, as well. I consider genetics a light switch on a dimmer. You may have the genetics to flip that light switch on, then the degree at which it expresses itself (the dimmer) is up to you and how you live.

Parents who are fat have fat kids for a couple of reasons. First, when parents are big, kids are big due to lifestyle. Intrauterine exposure to high amounts of insulin make for very large people (i.e., mom's lifestyle, diet, exercise patterns) which make the babies (someday to be adults) big. Second, kids tend to eat like their parents. If you grew up at McDonalds, you likely still eat there.

Epigenetics (meaning above genetics) is what controls your destiny. Epigenetics or things that change your genetic expression include:

- Stress
- Toxins
- Biotoxins
- Chemicals
- Nutrition/Diet/Food
- Lean mass vs. Fat mass

- Allergies
- Infections
- Hormones
- Inflammation
- Thoughts/Emotions

Does that list look or feel familiar? We have been discussing most of those items throughout the book.

Quick patient story. I have a wonderful late 30s, young woman patient, who is, by all standards, a big girl. She admittedly will never weigh less than 200 pounds. She came to me with two years of continual menstrual bleeding, fatigued all the time, and feeling like crap. She worked out twice a day, high intensity interval training, and crazy group classes at the local gym. She ate a very low-calorie diet, including bouts with the Human Chorionic Gonadotropin or hCG diet (would repeatedly lose 20 pounds and gain 25 pounds back within two weeks of stopping the hCG). Working with me, she has balanced her hormones (controlling her period, allowing her to get pregnant, etc.), exercises correctly now, and actually eats food. She has never felt better. She is very healthy by all medical standards (except her BMI, as she is a "naturally" big girl). She loves having me feel her biceps, and they are solid! Her quality of life is amazing (her words), but she will never be a fitness model, and that is OK with her. That, my friend, is a healthy woman—and something we should all strive for.

So, to answer your question, do you have a chance not to be fat and to feel good? Yes, you do. So work at it, just be real in your expectations.

**Can I maintain my look and feel good with this Fat to Fit to Fat *RecoverMe* program?**

Yes, you can. It will take some tweaking and continual adjustments, based on your schedule, family, vacations, job, sleep patterns, needs, etc. Hopefully, I have provided you with enough information to make it a lifelong program. If you get stuck due to an unexpected (or planned) variable, get in touch with me and I will do my best to help!

**What is the most toxic substance you can think of and one I should avoid at all costs?**

Bad relationships. Nothing more damaging, harmful, and soul wrenching. Don't ever forget that your mental and emotional health are vital for physical health. If you are in a bad or toxic relationship, be it with your spouse, boyfriend or girlfriend, boss, etc., get some help. You cannot expect anything I have discussed in this book to work unless you fix that toxic exposure.

**I am transitioning out of the MCD 5:2. What is the best way to decide what system or low carb/high carb day cycles to do next?**

In the summary chart, I gave you a few ideas, but the general concept is to go slow with it. Add high carb days based on your objective numbers (labs, body composition, etc.) and subjective feel (energy, sleep patterns, cognitive abilities, etc.).

I live by a 5:2 and have for 30 years. It works for me and my schedule. If I add an extra carb night in, I start getting a belly (bad genetics I have overcome with good epigenetics/lifestyle!). I have clients who live on a 2:1 and do great. You must find what works for you! I am, once again, happy to help if you need it.

**I have been following a personal trainer's suggestion on macros and exercise and have lost 10 pounds! I feel good overall, but no matter what I eat, I am getting bloated and feel I have stomach issues every day, except the weekends. Suggestions?**

First, you should know my opinion of "following macros"—it's bull-pucky! The type of food is just as important as the macros you consume. You are basically caught in the trap of modern thinking and your guts are telling you about it! The stress of the diet and exercise program your trainer has you on, combined with the Monday-Friday stress of your work week, play a toll on your guts due to elevated cortisol and the *type* of foods you have chosen to eat (basic flaw of macro worshipers)—that is why you are bloated all week but feel better on the weekends when you rest and I assume have a cheat meal (the answer was "yes" to the cheat meal).

This scenario plays out in many different presentations from gut issues, to brain issues, to sexual issues, to other hormonal issues—one of the reasons I wrote this book. This book is designed to make you aware of all the things that go wrong when you combine the stress of everyday living and add vigorous exercise and restrictive dieting to it. In one form or another, the Fat to Fit to Fat lifestyle will catch up to you if you are not aware of it.

**Are you a Republican or a Democrat?**

Neither. We need to start over in Washington.

**What if you are someone who does not like eating upon waking, but does not want to go as long as 8–10 hours before eating food? Could Track 2 be modified to eat 4–6 hours after waking?**

Well, anything is possible. If that style or timing works best for you, your situation, and your schedule, then do it. My basic point for suggesting each track was to give the reader a choice that would work around and/or fit their schedule the easiest. The goal is to eat appropriate foods, with minimal amounts being met, to allow for recovery and long-term maintenance. The goal is **NOT** to say one style of eating is better than another—there is no such thing as the perfect eating style. You must find one that works for you and your situation. One of the reasons there is so much "diet controversy" with all of the different eating suggestions out there, is that each limits itself to a protocol and if you fail that practice, you fail the diet. That's just dumb. Make your eating work for you, not against you!

**You mentioned that protein intake should be approximately 0.8 grams per pound of scale weight for women and 1 gram per pound of scale weight for men. What if someone is clearly overweight and weighs an excessive amount, would you still have them eat that many grams of protein, or is there a cutoff point? If they start to lose weight, will the protein grams decrease with the weight loss?**

Great question. This brings up a good point. Recall the five types of people I wrote this book for:

1. The man or woman who, at one time, trained their backside off and got into contest/stage shape, did a physique show, a bodybuilding show, or a fitness show and, following it, lost all their effort and cannot get that body back.

2. A person similar to those above who, no matter what they do, cannot get into bodybuilding, physique, or fitness shape.

3. The ex-college or professional athletes who finished playing their sport, lost all their lean mass, and replaced it with fat, against their will.

4. The people who cannot lose weight no matter how hard they try, including the good people who used to be thin/lean, but somehow 20 pounds snuck up on them.

5. The yo-yo dieter whose string finally broke.

This list did not, and purposefully, contain the morbidly obese defined by a BMI greater than 40 kg/m$^2$. Could someone with extreme weight issues use this book and do well? Most certainly—just applying some of the general principles outlined will help them lose fat.

The morbidly obese have several other issues to consider and I use different calculations when treating them. As a side note, and to answer the second part of your question—yes, as one loses weight, metabolism slows and it is a good idea to follow that change with food intake.

**What are the benefits of a protein powder having both whey hydrosolate and casein in it? You mentioned the benefits of each, but not if your protein powder has both.**

Protein powder with both casein and whey is a great option. Whey is quickly absorbed, casein is slowly absorbed, so the combo puts you somewhere in the middle. Mixed protein like this makes for a great post-workout meal as well. The combos are a little more expensive, but certainly a good option. Just remember what I stated earlier: casein protein causes allergy/sensitivity issues in some people, so know thyself.

**Doesn't less than 200 g of carbohydrates cause brain fog and fatigue? How can someone function on 35 g of carbohydrates per day, five consecutive days a week—especially with working out most days, and a vigorous schedule (or not)? You also mentioned to raise carb grams to 100 for women and 150 for men on the higher carb days (which still seems low), so how is that enough to restore glycogen stores after intake being so low for so many consecutive days?**

There is no magic number of carbohydrates to prevent brain fog. Carbohydrates are not essential nutrients, they are semi-essential. The more you exercise, the more you may benefit from them, but you can certainly live and function well without them. I love to tell people, "There is no such thing as a bad food, just bad diets." I am not criminalizing carbs here. I have found that lower carb diets help people obtain and maintain health and the physique they are after. Lower carb diets help the body rely on fat for energy utilization. Low carb diets tend to be low processed food diets—something huge for many people and likely one of the primary reasons so many people do so well with them.

Certainly, some people do better, feel better, and have less brain fog on a higher carbohydrate diet. Hopefully, they know that by now. If that is the case, increase the carbs in the diet, just stick to the other recommendations (eating style, what to do around eating, etc.) so your body can heal from the Fat to fit program.

As far as 100 or 150 grams of pure carbs filling glycogen stores, it does. Maybe not to the extent of *glycogen supercompensation* like I discuss in **Better Than Steroids**, but we are talking about a differ-ent group of people, in a very different circumstance. The 5:2 MCD discussed in Chapter 10 is designed to help you heal and get back on track to health and the body you want!

**I have always heard and read that delayed eating causes your body to store fat and slow metabolism when you finally do eat because it thinks it is protecting you for the next time it goes without food—basically, it won't trust you to feed it again for hours. Why doesn't this happen with the DET program? How does one not become hypoglycemic, as well? Does the supplement regimen prevent this?**

It takes roughly 96 hours for your body to go into slow everything down (metabolically) and start protecting and saving any food morsel that comes in as if we are starving. Think about it evolutionarily. Our great, great, great, great ancestors who roamed the plains, of what you now call home, were hunters and gatherers. If they missed a few meals, does it make sense that the body would shut down? No! The body speeds up and starts hunting and gathering to prevent death! With DET, we are talking a max of 16 hours without intake. Your body turns up the heat so you find some food after that fast. Not to mention if it fits your schedule, it will work for you just on that very fact alone!

Becoming hypoglycemic is a possibility for a rare few. Really—a rare few. The true medical diagnosis of "hypoglycemia" is associated with insulin use or a pancreatic tumor. Most who claim this condition have normal blood sugar—they have a sympathomimetic reaction to not eating, giving all the symptoms of hypoglycemia (e.g., anxiety, rapid heart rate, sweating, etc.).

Some hyper-insulin secretors, and even some with insulin resistance, might become this way, but that is why I suggest you check your blood sugars and/or drink some BCAA in water a few times during the fasting state.

**You mentioned that macrocounting is "bull-pucky"; is there ever a time and place for it?**

Let me clarify. Relying only on macros (or macronutrient counting) without being hyper-vigilant on the type of foods you eat, the timing of the foods you eat, and the hormonal response to the foods you eat, is silly. I suggest amounts in Chapter 10, but these are *minimal amounts*. Once you get an idea of that minimal amount, just eat every day and don't be so hung up on counting things out. Continually worrying about counting grams or calories is stressful and we are trying to lower your stress with this program, remember?

**Are there any added benefits to the temperature of the water I drink?**

Cold water is purported to require calories to heat up when you drink it. I think that is negligible. I like cold water, so I drink it. I have a good friend who likes room temperature water and he avoids ice in his drinks. My cold-water drink is not better than his, unless you want my opinion.

**What if you like the Track 1 way of eating, but still want a larger meal in the evening?**

I think that is fine, but you need to define "larger." If you tend to binge at night, when given the chance, there is a problem. If you have been following the program, the suggested supplements, etc., being ravenously hungry at night is less likely and eating a larger meal would be okay.

**The *RecoverMe* eating plan seems to be very low in calories (from looking at the sample menus) and restrictive on variety. How is that different from other low calorie diet programs?**

As discussed in Chapter 10, the amounts I suggest are *minimum amounts*. Eat some more if you are hungry. The ***RecoverMe*** plan is **NOT** restrictive—it is directional. In general, and if I were asked specifically about calories (as you just did), I am a low-calorie guy. I think there is enough good research out there on longevity and health in a low-calorie lifestyle vs. a Standard American Diet (SAD) lifestyle, that more people should pay attention to it. People tend to feel better eating the proper amounts of food vs. what they could eat just because it's there.

**I, personally, become physically sick or feel weird—for lack of a better description—when I eat a low-carb diet. How would the *RecoverMe* plan work for me when my body feels that way on low carbs?**

There are a couple of things you need to consider. Are you that way emotionally, or that way physiologically? Over time, on a lower carbohydrate intake eating plan, you should become better at utilizing fat as an energy source. If you are reading this book, there is an issue with your body and some of that might be that you are emotionally tied to carbs. For that reason, not a physiologic or metabolic reason, obtaining or getting back the body you want is more difficult. I would suggest a couple of things. We can run genetics on you and see if you are a better carb utilizer. If so, then we would focus on the types of carbs you eat, food timing, and the hormonal response to food, and design an eating plan specific to you. The majority of people reading this book will do very well with the 5:2 MCD I have set up, and I have thousands of case studies to prove it. If you do not do well with it, either come see me as a patient, or add a few more of the carbs I suggested in Chapter 10 to each meal and see how you do. If your body does not respond like you want, maybe we should talk?

**You mentioned that Track 1 eating is, "Better for people with diabetes, high cholesterol, etc." and Track 2 is "Better for people trying to lose as much fat as possible and still stay healthy." However, you stated that fitness stars, bodybuilders, etc. prefer more frequency of eating, as in Track 1. It seems as if Track 2 would be more beneficial to them for their fat loss goals. Would Track 2 be more effective for that population? What about for a fitness professional teaching multiple exercise classes a week (and sometimes multiple a day)—or even those gym rats who sometimes work out a few times a day (splitting up strength training and cardio).**

I describe Track 1 as "Better for people with diabetes and cholesterol issues," as that is what the medical literature has pointed out. These are lifestyle issues, so honestly, any improvements in eating will benefit these good people, Track 1 or Track 2. Bodybuilders who like to eat more frequently (the same goes for fitness professionals, or trainers/teachers), do well with it, as they are not likely suffering the ramifications of a Fat to Fit program yet (even though they are likely doing one). I know many bodybuilders who use DET dieting and do very well in their chosen sport. It is not as well-known as the classic five to seven meals a day eating plans found all over bodybuilding.com.

Over time, if your diet and exercise starts to catch up with you, you need to consider getting better, and that's when I would distinguish Track 1 or Track 2, based on your schedule and needs.

*I could have literally added a thousand more questions. I love questions. I get so excited to get email questions from readers and patients as it makes me think as well! If you have other questions or thoughts, please do not hesitate to email me! If I do not respond in 48 hours, send it again as it likely got buried!*

# APPENDIX I:
# THE WILLEY PRINCIPLE

In Chapter 2, I covered my issue with calories and why they are given so much credit for fat loss and fat gain. Years ago, I concluded that not all of this unfortunate misrepresentation was financial—there was a simple error in the original calculations. Several of the studies that define the fascination with calories today were done on lean, fit individuals. Could it be possible that calories-in-to-calories-out has more significance in lean people than in people with weight/fat issues?

Like every argument out there, there are extremes, but the answer usually lies somewhere in the middle. That is why I came up with The Willey Principle. It is simply a solution that lies in the middle of the "calories are all that matter" and "calories have nothing to do with it" arguments.

How would I prove this was the next question to come up? Setting up a study to demonstrate it would take time and money, both of which are limited in my life, so I went digging through patient files. I went through my own notes for bodybuilding show prep and I started to see a trend. I started to understand some, if not all, of the confusion as to the calories-in-to-calories-out question. I started to realize the reason for the discrepancy. In stepping back and looking at both sides, I finally realized something: Both sides are correct. That does not mean calories are the final solution or the end all, as you should now be aware from reading this book; it just means that calories play a role in fat/weight gain and loss, as has been suggested. As I mentioned in Chapter 2, studies have shown that there is an intra-human variance of fat storage (up to a ten-fold difference) in response to caloric consumption. Maybe a lot of this has to do with the starting point of the weight/fat loss?

The Willey Principle states:

- **Dependency on caloric load is greater the leaner you get.**

Simply put, the bigger you are, the less you should worry about calories-in-to-calories-out. The smaller or leaner you are, the more calories-in-to-calories-out comes into play. To add a little more detail to the theory, *direct* caloric counting and portion sizing become more essential the leaner one gets. If you are extremely large, just learning how to eat with a focus on higher quality foods will start the weight loss process. Get your HPA Axis lined up, get your hormones balanced, fix your gut, remove yourself from toxins and environmental hazards, and consider being more meticulous about calories as you get leaner.

Anyone and everyone in the dietary world would be of the same opinion that larger people have an easier time losing weight at first, operative words being "at first!" There are several reasons for this, including the fact that larger people actually have faster metabolisms than smaller people. As a result, *any* change in the larger person's eating habits, caloric load (direct or indirect), will assist in weight/fat loss.

People come to me all the time for that last 10 or 20 pounds they cannot get off, and to get it off, (after applying the principles outlined in this book) I play with their caloric intake. When a larger person comes in needing to lose a few hundred pounds, however, I do not initially restrict their calories. I give them the principles outlined here and they do wonderfully, no matter whether they are tracking their calories or not. Remember: too large a caloric deficit is a Fat to Fit concept.

This brings up another very important concept closely related to The Willey Principle. It is called The P ratio, or Partitioning Ratio. This basically means the leaner you are, the more lean muscle mass you will lose with dieting. The fatter you are, the more fat you will lose with dieting. So when skinny people diet, they lose muscle, whereas when people with more body fat diet, they lose more body fat (to a point). The morbidly obese can tolerate lower calories than the moderately obese, with greater retention of fat free mass. This is why The Willey Principle works. If you maintain the style of eating outlined here, you will have an easier time maintaining weight/fat loss. It will also give you some direction to go from your current starting point (something that changes every time you measure).

# APPENDIX II: PROTEIN SOURCES WITH GRAMS PER SERVING SIZE

| PROTEIN SOURCE | SERVING SIZE | GRAMS PROTEIN |
|---|---|---|
| 1% COTTAGE CHEESE | 1 CUP | 24 |
| 2% COTTAGE CHEESE (LOW FAT) | 1 CUP | 30 |
| COTTAGE CHEESE (FAT FREE) | 1 CUP | 28 |
| COTTAGE CHEESE DRY CURD | 1 CUP | 24 |
| BASS, FRESHWATER, DRY HEAT | 4 OZ | 28 |
| BASS, STRIPED, DRY HEAT | 4 OZ | 25 |
| CHEDDAR, SHREDDED, FAT FREE | 0.25 CUP | 10 |
| CHEDDAR, SHREDDED, 94% FAT FREE | 0.25 CUP | 8 |
| CHEESE, COLBY/MOZZARELLA | 4 OZ | 28 |
| MOZZARELLA SHREDDED, FAT FREE | 0.25 CUP | 9 |
| CHICKEN BREAST (HORMEL/CAN) | 1 CAN | 30 |
| CHICKEN BREAST (SKINLESS) | 4 OZ | 26 |
| CHICKEN (LEG W/ SKIN & BONE) | 1 | 30 |
| CHICKEN (THIGH W/ SKIN & BONE) | 1 | 16 |
| CHICKEN (LEG & THIGH W/ SKIN & BONE) | 1 | 45 |
| COD, ATLANTIC, DRY HEAT | 4 OZ | 25 |
| CRAB, ALASKA KING, MOIST HEAT | 4 OZ | 23 |
| CRAB, BLUE, MOIST HEAT | 4 OZ | 23 |
| EGG WHITE | 3 | 11 |
| EGG, WHOLE | 3 | 20 |
| EGG BEATERS | 1 CUP | 24 |
| FLOUNDER, DRY HEAT | 4 OZ | 28 |
| HADDOCK, DRY HEAT | 4 OZ | 28 |
| HALIBUT, DRY HEAT | 4 OZ | 31 |
| HAM 96% FAT FREE | 4 OZ | 18 |
| HAM, DARK MEAT, CANNED | 4 OZ | 20 |
| HAMBURGER, (10% FAT) | 4 OZ | 29 |
| HAMBURGER, (15% FAT) | 4 OZ | 29 |
| HAMBURGER, (20% FAT) | 4 OZ | 20 |
| HAMBURGER, (27% FAT) | 4 OZ | 27 |
| LAMB, SHOULDER | 4 OZ | 14 |
| LOBSTER, NORTHERN, MOIST HEAT | 4 OZ | 23 |
| MAHI MAHI | 4 OZ | 21 |
| ORANGE ROUGHY, DRY HEAT | 4 OZ | 21 |
| PERCH, DRY HEAT | 4 OZ | 28 |
| PERCH, OCEAN/ATLANTIC, DRY HEAT | 4 OZ | 28 |
| PORK, SIRLOIN, LEAN W/ FAT | 4 OZ | 25 |
| SALMON, ATLANTIC, DRY HEAT | 4 OZ | 29 |
| SHRIMP, MOIST HEAT | 4 OZ | 24 |

| PROTEIN SOURCE | SERVING SIZE | | GRAMS PROTEIN |
|---|---|---|---|
| STEAK, BOTTOM ROUND | 4 | OZ | 36 |
| STEAK, BRISKET (FLAT HALF) | 4 | OZ | 36 |
| STEAK, CHUCK, ARM | 4 | OZ | 37 |
| STEAK, CHUCK, BLADE | 4 | OZ | 35 |
| STEAK, EYE ROUND | 4 | OZ | 33 |
| STEAK, FLANK | 4 | OZ | 31 |
| STEAK, NEW YORK STRIP | 4 | OZ | 30 |
| STEAK, PORTERHOUSE | 4 | OZ | 32 |
| STEAK, RIB EYE | 4 | OZ | 32 |
| STEAK, ROUND TIP | 4 | OZ | 35 |
| STEAK, SHANK (CROSSCUTS) | 4 | OZ | 39 |
| STEAK, T-BONE | 4 | OZ | 32 |
| STEAK, TENDERLOIN | 4 | OZ | 31 |
| STEAK, TOP LOIN | 4 | OZ | 32 |
| STEAK, TOP ROUND | 4 | OZ | 36 |
| STEAK, TOP SIRLOIN | 4 | OZ | 35 |
| STEAK, TYSON SEASONED BEEF STRIPS | 4 | OZ | 27 |
| TROUT, DRY HEAT | 4 | OZ | 31 |
| TUNA, LOW SODIUM, CANNED | 1 | CAN | 39 |
| TUNA, WATER, CANNED | 1 | CAN | 32 |
| TUNA, WHITE / LO SALT, CAN (1 CAN / 5 OZ) | 1 | CAN | 37 |
| TUNA, WHITE, CAN (1 CAN / 5 OZ) | 1 | CAN | 40 |
| TUNA, FILLET/STEAK | 4 | OZ | 32 |
| TURKEY BREAST (SKINLESS) | 4 | OZ | 32 |
| TURKEY BREAST (CANNED) | 1 | CAN | 28 |
| TURKEY BREAST/OVEN ROAST - 89% FF | 4 | OZ | 16 |
| VENISON / ANTELOPE | 4 | OZ | 34 |
| WALLEYE | 4 | OZ | 28 |
| ALMONDS | 1 | OZ | 6 |
| BEANS, PINTO (DRY) | 0.25 | CUP | 10 |
| BROCCOLI, FRESH | 1 | CUP | 3 |
| CHICKPEAS / GARBANZO BEANS | 0.25 | CUP | 10 |
| KIDNEY BEANS (DRY) | 0.25 | CUP | 11 |
| LENTIL (COOKED) | 0.5 | CUP | 9 |
| MILK (2%) | 8 | OZ | 10 |
| MILK (1%) | 8 | OZ | 9 |
| MILK, SKIM | 8 | OZ | 8 |
| SOYBEANS (BOILED) | 0.5 | CUP | 11 |
| YOGURT, FAT FREE | 8 | OZ | 11 |
| YOGURT, NONFAT, LITE | 8 | OZ | 8 |
| YOGURT, FAT FREE, LITE | 6 | OZ | 6 |
| YOGURT, YOPLAIT ORIGINAL/99% FAT FREE | 6 | OZ | 6 |

# APPENDIX III: MEDITATION AND SAUNA USE

## Meditation

As you are healing, one thing you may really want to consider is meditation. I am certainly no expert on the topic, having only recently started it on a regular basis myself. But I can tell you, the benefits are noticeable from day one and improve additive from then forward!

Meditation changes the brain. Literally changes the brain. It causes more neurons to grow and connect, increases the size of certain areas of the brain that serve to help with attention, awareness, visual processing. It also changes the lower portion of the hippocampus and helps modify its role in releasing cortisol under stressful situations.

It causes parts of the brain to get smaller, such as the amygdala I discussed earlier when we reviewed the role of stress and cortisol on the brain. A smaller amygdala means you are less likely to freak out about things when something goes wrong.

In my goal to keep this short, let me list a few of the benefits of meditation and I think you will quickly see how it will fit in to your recovery program from your Fat to Fit plan:

- **Improved mood**
- **Calming effect**
- **Lowers stress**
- **Improves happiness**
- **Increases pain thresholds**
- **Improves focus and attention**
- **Increases self-awareness**
- **Lowers blood pressure and heart rate**
- **Helps to regulate blood sugar and insulin**
- **Improves the immune system**
- **Increases neuroplasticity and heals the brain, making your brain "younger"**

I would consider meditation an essential part of a *RecoverMe* program as any health concern, fatigue issue, quality of life issues, etc., can be greatly improved if you just take a few minutes each day and meditate.

A simple and very cheap way to get involved with daily meditation is have the good people at www.calm.com guide you. This web site provides a lot of great information, techniques, and help to get you on a path to health via meditation. There are actual sessions you can do via apps and the web and a few only take 10 min a day! For $12.99 a month or $60.00 for a year, you can have your own meditation coach. Well worth the small fee as meditation should certainly be part of your life.

PS: I am not paid by calm.com; I just think it is a good and helpful site.

## Infrared Sauna

"Heat treatments" have been used for thousands of years by almost all civilizations. They have been primarily known to help with relaxation and detoxification. Current research is pointing to all sorts of benefits from sauna use, in particular, infrared saunas. Infrared saunas have the benefit of heating the skin to cause sweating, but does not warm the air around you. This allows for lower temperature treatments for those who may not tolerate steam or dry air saunas. It also allows for in home use, as infrared "boxes" are fairly inexpensive and safe for use.

How saunas work exactly can be debated, however the research appears to show that they act at the cellular level, causing an increase in metabolism via activation of the cell membranes and mitochondria. They also cause profuse sweating and thereby removal of cellular waste (detoxification).

The benefits of infrared saunas in relation to healing from your previous health or body attainment program include the following:

- **Muscle and joint relaxation and healing**
- **Pain relief**
- **Detoxification**
- **Help with insomnia**
- **Help with depression**
- **Cardiac health/healing including lowering blood pressure, lowering LDL, and increasing HDL**
- **Improved hormonal activity**
- **Less fatigue**
- **Improved ability to relax**

- **Skin cleansing**
- **Improved exercise capacity**

I use my infrared sauna at least three times a week. It makes a noticeable difference in overall quality of life and energy levels. I would highly encourage you to consider one either for home use or find a local spa or health club with one. Wet saunas probably do a lot of good as well, but the research I reviewed before purchasing one myself was all on infrared saunas.

# CONTACT INFORMATION

Warren Willey
Email: doc@drwilley.com
Web sites:
www.drwilley.com
www.chewitkids.org

*Dr. Willey lives in Southeast Idaho with his lovely bride and three kids. He has been blessed to serve his community by overseeing a large medical practice and a great team of 10 providers. A large percentage of his patients travel in from out of town to consult with him, particularly the list of people he mentioned in the book (professional athletes, bodybuilders and fitness competitors, people stuck in their health attempts, people with chronic disease who want an outside opinion, etc.). He has a patient list that extends all over the United States and the world. He enjoys being outside as often as possible and his favorite drug is weightlifting.*

# index

## symbols

5-HTP  316
8-hydroxydeoxyguanosine (8-OHdG)  163
28-day hormone tests for women  171

## a

AAS  19, 99, 104, 105, 106, 131, 144, 145, 150, 153, 182, 183, 287, 314
Acetyl-L-Carnitine  190, 283
ACTH  75, 133, 135
adiponectin  25, 50, 138, 141, 142, 154, 155, 157, 241, 249, 278
Adiponectin  25, 154, 155, 249
adrenal gland  75, 133, 207
Advanced Lipid Testing  173
aldosterone  77
Allostatic Load  69, 70
Alpha Lipoic Acid (ALA)  289
Ambien (Zolpidem)  320
amphetamines  99
amygdala  80, 355
anabolic  19, 20, 21, 80, 89, 104, 105, 144, 153, 170, 171, 182, 238, 250, 252, 294, 306
Anabolic/androgenic steroids  99
anabolic to catabolic ratio  170
Anavar  36, 42, 105
Antidepressants  45
anti-inflammatories  183, 191
antioxidants  16, 101, 161, 183, 184, 187, 191, 193, 241, 290
antipsychotics  45, 310
Arsenic  166
At Home Labs  168

autoimmune diseases  91, 93
autonomic nervous system  76

## B

Bariatric  22, 23
BCAA  34, 185, 253, 272, 342
Beetroot  191
Berberine  283
Beta 3 receptors  107
Beta-alanine  190
Better Than Steroids  245
bisphenol A (BPA)  166
bisphenol B (BPB)  166
bloating  192, 112, 158, 185, 253
blood brain barrier (BBB)  111
Blood Pressure  169
bodybuilding  xiv, 5, 33, 35, 37, 57, 73, 174, 230, 231, 248, 339, 345, 347
body comp  61, 245
Bonito Proteins  186
Boswellia  282
Bowel Bollix  93, 130, 134, 158
brain hormones  39, 62, 65, 88, 96, 102, 138, 143, 144, 146, 312

## c

Calm Energy  282
calories  3, 13, 15, 16, 17, 18, 19, 20, 22, 23, 24, 26, 30, 31, 41, 46, 52, 57, 58, 84, 85, 87, 88, 89, 96, 99, 106, 109, 111, 116, 117, 118, 122, 145, 229, 230, 231, 233, 236, 249, 250, 251, 266, 269, 271, 326, 333, 342, 343, 347, 348
can be seen on a functional MRI  81
cancer  24, 122, 154, 159, 163, 243, 267, 314, 327, 333
carbs  31, 84, 87, 89, 95, 168, 174, 201, 235, 238, 240 249, 250, 254, 255, 257, 258, 260, 271, 273,

306, 316, 341, 343, 344
Chemistry Panel 131
chronic fatigue syndrome 80, 134, 186
Chronic stress 76, 149, 151
Clen 107, 109
Clenbuterol 36, 42, 107
Cognitive behavior therapy 321
Complete Blood Count (CBC) 131
comprehensive gut analysis 46
Contemporary Diet and Exercise Recommendations 49
CoQ10 97, 194
Cordyceps sinensis 287
cortisol 12, 39, 44, 46, 50, 60, 69, 70 74, 75, 76, 77, 79, 80, 88, 92, 118, 130, 132, 133, 134, 135, 136, 138, 141, 142, 143, 144, 147, 148, 149, 152, 157, 158, 160, 171, 179, 183, 192, 194, 198, 237, 243, 249, 251, 262, 282, 287, 299, 307, 308, 309, 311, 312, 316, 317, 330, 338
CRH 75, 133, 308
Cytomel 80, 146, 147

## d

Delayed Eating Techniques 238, 244
depressed 38, 49, 61, 88, 269
DET 238, 244, 245, 256, 272, 273, 341, 342, 344
DHEA 46, 50, 62, 133, 135, 136, 141, 142, 143, 150, 151, 171, 312
diagnosis 21, 112, 113, 123, 129, 155, 156, 196, 342
diet xiv, 4, 5,6, 7, 8, 9, 12, 13, 14, 16, 17, 18, 24, 26, 29, 31, 34, 35, 37, 39, 40, 42, 46, 48,, 52, 53, 54, 58, 66, 69, 70, 71, 74, 76, 77, 78, 79, 81, 83, 84, 85, 87, 88, 89, 90, 91, 92, 94, 95, 96, 99, 100, 101, 102, 103, 104, 105

107, 108, 109, 110, 112, 113, 115, 116, 117, 121, 122, 123, 124, 125, 128, 129, 130, 131, 132, 134, 138, 140, 141, 143, 144, 145, 146, 148, 149, 150, 151, 152, 153, 157, 158, 160, 161, 163, 164, 165, 166, 169, 172, 173, 174, 175, 180, 181, 182, 183, 184, 186, 189, 190, 191, 192, 195, 196, 229, 230, 231, 232, 233, 237, 240, 242, 243, 247, 248, 249, 251 255, 262, 265, 266, 268, 269, 281, 283, 284, 298, 299, 300, 310, 325, 326, 327, 328, 329, 330, 333, 335, 336, 338, 339, 341, 343
Digestion/Absorption Indicators 159
DIM 241, 242, 261, 288
diurnal salivary cortisol 317
D-ribose 186
drugs 7, 16, 20, 22, 33, 37, 38, 39, 69, 70, 77, 80, 93, 94, 96, 99, 102, 103, 104, 105, 106, 107, 107, 109, 113, 123, 131, 142, 144, 146, 147, 150, 155, 158, 161, 165, 249, 296, 272, 273, 280, 291, 293, 301, 304, 307, 308, 309, 310, 312, 318, 319, 332

## e

E2 152, 153
Electrolytes 132
endotoxemia 78
environment 22, 25, 26, 66, 92, 133, 135, 139, 142, 173, 297, 301, 302, 303, 305, 306, 335
Estradiol 152, 153
Estrogen 62
Eurycoma longifolia 287
exercise xv, 1, 2, 3, 4, 5, 6, 7, 12, 13, 14, 15, 16, 17, 18, 19, 20, 24, 26,

29, 32, 39, 46, 48, 50, 51, 52, 53, 54, 58, 60, 62, 63, 64, 66, 69, 70, 71, 73, 74, 75, 80, 81, 103, 104, 109, 110, 101, 102, 103, 104, 105, 106, 107, 108, 109, 110, 112, 113, 119, 121, 122, 123, 124, 125, 128, 129, 130, 131, 132, 134, 138, 140, 141, 143, 144, 146, 148, 149, 150, 151, 152, 153, 155, 157, 158, 159, 160, 161, 163, 164, 165, 166, 169, 172, 173, 175, 178, 179, 180, 181, 182, 183, 184, 186, 189, 190, 191, 192, 194, 195, 196, 197, 198, 199, 200, 201, 202, 203, 204, 205, 206, 207, 208, 209, 210, 213, 214, 216, 218, 225, 226, 229, 237, 238, 240, 243, 247, 249, 251, 253, 257, 261, 262, 265, 266, 268, 272, 281, 283, 284, 287, 288, 293, 298, 299, 300, 301, 307, 310, 311, 312, 316, 325, 326, 327, 328, 329, 330, 331, 333, 335, 337, 338, 340, 344, 346

Exogenous 112

## f

Fasting glucose 168
Fat xvi, 4, 24, 25, 26, 38, 40, 44, 46, 47, 49, 50, 53, 59, 60, 62, 64, 76, 84, 88, 92, 93, 95, 104, 111, 115, 116, 117, 125, 132, 148, 153, 157, 162, 164, 165, 168, 170, 173, 177, 182, 184, 186, 188, 193, 195, 196, 200, 201, 208, 225, 233, 243, 244, 249, 250, 251, 254, 256, 257, 261, 262, 265, 270, 277, 278, 279, 280, 282, 283, 284, 287, 288, 290, 294, 297, 298, 300, 308, 312, 317, 320, 321, 325, 326, 327, 328, 329, 330, 334, 335, 336, 338, 341, 344, 351
fatigue 4, 6, 8, 29, 48, 57, 65, 76, 77, 80, 81, 96, 111, 117, 134, 186, 189, 190, 272, 290, 295, 310, 340, 356, 357
Follicle-Stimulating Hormone 144
Food Sensitivity Testing 160
Food Timing 20
free radical 93
FSH 62, 144
Full-Body CrossFit Program 201

## g

Gamma-glutamyl transferase (GGT) 164
gastroenterologist 43, 90, 159
Gastrointestinal 84, 90
Genetic Testing 172
glucagon 18, 138, 141, 142, 249, 250, 256
Green tea 191
gut bacteria 22, 91, 92, 93
Gut bugs 160
Gut Immunology 159
Gut Integrity Markers 160
gut test 46, 50

## h

Hawthorn Berry 189
heart disease 24, 118, 122, 154, 161, 162, 163, 164, 186, 243, 283
heart rate variability (HRV) 76
Heart Rate Variability (HRV) 170
Holiday and Vacation Meal Planning and Eating 259
Holy Basil 194

Hormonal 84, 85, 129, 138, 143
Hormonal Havoc 129, 138
hormone 12, 18, 21, 23, 39, 45, 46, 50, 52, 53, 54, 57, 58, 60, 65, 66, 70, 74, 75, 77, 79, 80, 85, 86, 87, 88, 90, 103, 104, 105, 109, 110, 111, 113, 115, 129, 132, 133, 140, 141, 142, 143, 144, 145, 147, 148, 149, 150, 152, 153, 155, 157, 171, 183, 184, 185, 193, 196, 199, 206, 249, 250, 254, 256, 267, 278, 284, 288, 289, 294, 297, 299, 307, 308, 309, 310, 312, 314, 315
Hormones 45, 85, 110, 135, 139, 144, 182, 284, 297, 336
hot flashes 52, 54
HPA axis 49, 75, 133, 134, 135, 233, 262, 299, 312
HPA Axis Adversity 74, 129, 130, 132
hungry 13, 34, 40, 87, 156, 233, 247, 251, 343
hypothalamus 75, 80, 133, 134, 142, 308

## i

IGF-1 104, 153, 154, 250, 256
immune 70, 75, 87, 90, 92, 93, 116, 133, 134, 145, 146, 147, 160, 161, 284, 287, 294, 297, 356
inflammation 70, 91, 151, 152, 154, 159, 163, 183, 239, 241, 243, 248, 249, 250, 290
Insomnia 70
insulin 4, 18, 21, 86, 102, 104, 121, 122, 134, 138, 141, 142, 145, 150, 151, 153, 154, 155, 156, 157, 164, 166, 168, 169, 172, 183, 188, 206, 241, 249, 250, 256, 262, 263, 278, 281, 284, 305, 306, 314, 335, 342, 356

Insulin 21, 50, 70, 86, 153, 155, 156
irritable bowel 93, 134, 159

## k

Kombucha 46

## L

leaky gut 93, 148, 156, 160, 166
leptin 25, 44, 50, 87, 88, 89, 90, 121, 138, 141, 147, 148, 156, 157, 206, 249, 250, 256, 294
Leptin 87, 88, 89, 142, 156, 157, 249, 294
L-Glutamine 284
LH 62, 133, 144, 145
Lipopolysaccharide 79
low carb 40, 248, 249, 250, 251, 272, 343
LPS 79, 164, 194
L-Taurine 284
L-Theanine 46, 282, 315
L-Tyrosine 289
Lunesta (Eszopiclone) 320
Luteinizing Hormone 144

## m

magnesium 63, 95, 197, 125, 132, 169, 188, 189, 195, 278, 281, 317, 330
Magnesium 188
meditation 355
melatonin 75, 171, 289, 300, 304, 307, 308, 315, 316
Melatonin 289, 315
menopausal 143, 232, 266
Menopause 52, 53
menstrual cycle 13, 43, 49, 143, 144, 152, 180, 314

mental health  123
messengers  45, 85, 86, 139, 182
Metabolic Indicators  160
metabolic rate  12, 18, 109, 115
Mixed Tocotrienols/Tocopherols(Vitamin E)  188
MPO  163, 164
Multivitamin with minerals  282

## n

N-AcetylCystine (NAC)  283
Negative 5  206
neurotransmitters  44, 96, 108, 141, 142, 143, 167, 196, 230, 243, 289, 294, 310, 311
night sweats  52, 54
Nutritional  84, 100, 124
nutritional deficiencies  92, 101, 158

## o

Omega-3 Fatty Acids  290
One-hour post-prandial glucose  168
overexercising  15, 16, 56, 92, 111, 112, 125, 129, 142, 146, 147, 154, 155, 156, 161, 165, 167, 170, 179, 195, 197, 226, 241, 243, 245, 266, 273, 278, 283, 289, 296, 299, 311
Oxandrolone  105
oxidative stress  2, 49, 53, 81, 161, 162, 163, 164, 191, 200, 230, 233, 248, 258, 274, 283, 284, 301, 333

## P

parasympathetic  78
paraventricular nucleus  77
Passionflower  284
Pattern 1  295, 299, 311, 312, 313, 316, 317, 318
Pattern 2  295, 299, 300, 317, 318, 319, 320, 321
Pea-based protein powder  185
peptides  104, 186
pH  164, 169, 187, 242, 282, 330
Phentermine  41, 108, 109
Phosphatidylserine  287
Phosphorylated Serine  46, 317
phthalates  166
Post-Workout Meal  192
Pre- and Post-Workout Meals  183
Prebiotics  93
probiotic  93, 160
progesterone  50, 62, 63, 144, 148, 149, 186, 171, 314
Progesterone  148, 149, 313, 314
progestin  52, 314
prohormone  34, 103
Prohormones  103
Prolactin  145
Protein  96, 185, 193, 250, 270, 340, 351
Pulse  169

## r

Rachel McLish  47, 48, 51
RBC Mg+  62, 63, 132, 189, 278, 281, 330
RecoverMe  50, 51, 54, 60, 76, 100, 122, 123, 124, 125, 130, 131, 136, 158, 168, 177, 179, 182, 183, 184, 186, 187, 193, 195, 196, 197, 198, 200, 201, 214, 226, 227, 229, 232, 233, 237, 239, 241, 245, 246, 247, 250, 251, 254, 256, 257, 258, 259, 260, 261, 262, 267, 270, 272, 275, 277, 280, 291, 293, 295, 297, 301, 306, 308, 321, 326, 327, 329, 330, 333, 334,

336, 343, 356
Relora 46, 282
Resistant Starch 187
Reverse Dieting 42, 230
Reverse T3 81
Rhodiola 316
Round Up 167
rT3 81, 82, 88, 148

## s

SARMs 104
sdLDL 173
sex 4, 25, 29, 43, 44, 49, 53, 54, 65, 70, 71, 82, 83, 103, 138, 141, 142, 151, 157, 196, 207, 243, 244, 302
sexual function 37, 43, 89, 138, 151, 152
SHBG 82, 149, 150, 288
sleep 1, 4, 15, 25, 26, 35, 38, 39, 46, 52, 54, 55, 60, 71, 77, 70, 91, 92, 96, 102, 111, 123, 132, 149, 152, 182, 232, 269, 272, 274, 289, 293, 294, 295, 296, 297, 298, 299, 300, 301, 302, 303, 304, 305, 306, 307, 308, 309, 310, 311, 312, 314, 315, 316, 317, 318, 320, 321, 326, 337

social media 3, 48, 51, 122
SOD1 and SOD2 163
Speed Sets 216
Stress 77, 130, 133, 161, 335
stress levels 39, 69, 170, 199
supplement 34, 35, 39, 41, 51, 100, 102, 105, 113, 117, 125, 132, 160, 190, 191, 195, 240, 241, 242, 250, 254, 260, 261, 278, 279, 280, 282, 283, 287, 288, 290, 291, 301, 317, 330, 341
supplementation 94, 195, 118, 301, 311
suprachiasmatic nucleus (SCN) 77
sympathetic 77, 78, 96, 107, 108, 169, 189, 249, 284, 298, 307

## t

T3 18, 50, 81, 82, 88, 109, 110, 111, 146, 147, 148
T4 81, 110, 111, 146, 147, 148
Taurine 189
testosterone 50, 62, 63, 65, 81, 82, 88, 89, 99, 103, 112, 141, 144, 149, 150, 151, 152, 157, 171, 182, 249, 250, 256, 262, 278, 287, 288
Testosterone 36, 81, 88, 89, 102, 151, 152
testosterone/cortisol ratio 82
The Environmental Working Group 333
The Free Window 256
The lifestyle hormones 86
The National Weight Control Registry 14, 15
The Poop Test 159
Thermogenics 101
The T Club 112, 249
The Under-Recovery Syndrome 166
The Z Diet 84
The Z-Drugs (Nonbenzodiazepine Hypnotics) 302
thyroid 18, 25, 44, 49, 50, 62, 63, 65, 81, 82, 86, 88, 99, 109, 110, 111, 112, 133, 134, 138, 141, 142, 145, 146, 147, 148, 153, 157, 160, 171, 180, 196, 207, 236, 249, 254, 256, 262, 269, 289, 290
Thyroid Peroxidase Antibody 147
thyroid-stimulating hormone (TSH) 81, 110, 111, 133
Toxins 25, 165, 166, 284, 335
Toxin Trouble 130, 164
Track 1 244, 246, 247, 248, 255, 261,

    262, 268, 270, 271, 343, 344, 345
Track 2  244, 245, 246, 247, 248, 255,
    261, 265, 267, 271, 272, 273,
    306, 338, 344, 345
Triiodothyronine  109, 146, 147

## u

under-recovery  62, 170
Urinary hormone metabolites  171

## v

very low-calorie diets  115
very low energy diets  115
visceral fat  26, 121, 154, 169
vitamin  94, 95, 100, 188, 194, 281,
    288, 290, 308
Vitamin C  187, 281
Vitamin D3  288

## W

workouts  34, 40, 42, 46, 55, 57, 59, 82

## x

Xenoestrogens  166
Xyrem (Sodium Oxybate)  321

## z

Zinc/Magnesium/B6  317